# FAT
# LOSS
## REVOLUTION

## LOVE AND PRAISE FOR FAT LOSS REVOLUTION

If you want to know the truth about losing weight, and what you absolutely must do to improve your health, this is the book for you. Paula reveals the facts in a compelling and insightful way. This invaluable book belongs on the bookshelf of anyone who wants the truth to experience optimal health and permanent fat loss.

> **J.J. Virgin, CNS, CHFS**
> *New York Times* bestselling author of *The Virgin Diet*

Paula Owens is one of my go-to experts when it comes to nutrition, fitness, hormones and lifestyle for women. I first met Paula at a seminar close to 15 years ago and ever since she has continued to invest in ongoing education, seeking out experts to learn from, and applying what she knows with herself and her clients. She is one of THE MOST KNOWLEDGEABLE people I know when it comes to fat loss for women. How you look on the outside is a reflection of how healthy you are on the inside, which is exactly why Paula's approach works. The information in her book leads to a healthy body inside and out, with balanced hormones, optimal health and looking fabulous! She covers EVERYTHING in this book, giving you her secrets, lists, recipes, workouts and tips to guarantee you find your own hot and healthy body.

> **Rachel Cosgrove,** Bestselling author of *The Female Body Breakthrough* and co-owner of Results Fitness

Paula Owens has written one of the most comprehensive resources for anyone looking to shed fat pounds. Not only does she cover diet and exercise, but she also guides you down the rabbit hole of those hidden factors contributing to weight gain including food sensitivities, toxins, mindset, and even parasites! This one is a winner.

> **Sean Croxton,** Underground Wellness and author of *The Dark Side of Fat Loss*

Move over Dr. Oz....here is Paula Owens with the absolute truth about long-term fat loss and healthy weight loss. If you wish to get in shape just follow the book's instructions to the tee. This book should be in every home library.

**Eric Serrano, M.D.**

---

Paula knows how to get results! If you have tried other diet books and found them lacking, fear not, you will love the *Fat Loss Revolution.*

**Robb Wolf**

*New York Times* bestselling author of *The Paleo Solution*

---

Teach a girl to diet and she'll always fail; teach a girl to lean out through hormonal balance and detoxification and she'll be lean for life! I truly love this book and think it's so damn smart. The *Fat Loss Revolution* is THE go-to resource for the woman who wants to settle the score between herself and her body--for good. Paula gives you the straight dope on clean eating and fat-burning exercises that will help you shed unwanted pounds and have the body you never thought possible, no matter what your age or your starting point. She is living proof it can be done!

**Esther Blum, MS, RD, CDN, CNS**, Bestselling author of *Eat, Drink, and Be Gorgeous* and *Cavewomen Don't Get Fat*

---

While most of the mainstream dieting world is still obsessively (and incorrectly) focused on cutting calories as a means for producing weight loss, Paula offers an alternative theory backed by the very latest science showing that what you really want is fat loss. And the best way to make this happen is to become educated about the vital role the proper balance of hormones play, discovering the foods that will control these hormones naturally and having an effective plan to make it happen for you. *Fat Loss Revolution* is the first step in changing your life forever!

**Jimmy Moore**, author of *21 Life Lessons From Livin' La Vida Low-Carb*

---

## MORE LOVE AND PRAISE FOR FAT LOSS REVOLUTION

Paula has hit a home run again with *Fat Loss Revolution.* Paula designed my personal diet and conditioning regimes and I can tell you they absolutely work.

I'm currently 74 years of age. I have been following the information in the book since being introduced to Paula more than 20 years ago and my weight has not varied more than 2-4 pounds during that period. Muscle increase has been difficult for me because of a three year bout with polio when I was a child, however, using her system I have not lost muscle mass and this is not bad for someone who could not walk for more than three years.

Employ the sage advice found in this book and I can assure you will prevent disease, gain muscle and lose fat.

**Harry O. Eidenier. Jr. Ph.D.**
Director of D.S.D. International, Ltd.

Paula so eloquently describes the amount of awareness required for good health in this book. You cannot lose fat nor have a hot body without overall good health. She is beginning an evolution of *truth* in wellness care – for life. She educates readers on how the complex interaction of body systems, hormones, chemicals and lifestyle relate to fat loss. This book is a wakeup call to the amount of self-awareness that is necessary to create well-being.

**Theresa Ramsey, N.M.D.**

Paula Owens not only understands how fat loss works, she explains it in easy-to-understand terms that will make perfect sense and leave you excited to get started immediately. Do what she says for 12 weeks and you'll be thanking yourself forever.

**Mark Sisson**, author of the *Primal Blueprint* and publisher of MarksDailyApple.com

# FAT
# LOSS
## REVOLUTION

12 Weeks to a
Hot 'n Healthy
Body at Any Age

# PAULA OWENS

**ISBN-10:** 0615654207

**ISBN-13:** 978-0-615-65420-1

The information presented in this publication is based on the training and professional experience of the author and is for educational purposes only. It is not intended to diagnose illness nor prescribe treatment nor replace a doctor's treatment. Rather, the material presented in this book is designed to be used in cooperation with your nutritional health professional. Following tips or recommendations does not ensure that you will be healthy. Your health is the result of many factors, some of which are not yet fully understood. It is important that you rely on the personal advice of a healthcare professional to advise you on your specific situation. Proper laboratory and clinical monitoring is essential to achieve the goals of finding safe and natural treatments. Should you use the information on your own, you are prescribing for yourself, which is your constitutional right. The author and the publisher hereby disclaim any and all liability and responsibility resulting from injuries or damage caused by following any recommendations contained in this book.

The workouts and other health-related activities described in this book were developed by the author and are to be used as an adjunct to improved strengthening, conditioning, health and fitness. These programs may not be appropriate for everyone. All individuals and especially those who suffer from disease or are recovering from an injury of any sort should consult their physician regarding the advisability of undertaking any of the activities suggested in these programs. The author and the publisher are neither responsible nor liable for any harm or injury resulting from the programs or the use of the exercises or exercise devices described herein.

# CONTENTS

---

# PREFACE

After writing and publishing my first book, *The Power of 4,* I had no intention of writing another book. However, as time passed I continued to experience a deep, burning desire to share more of my knowledge and passion for nutrition, fitness and health. This book is an informative compilation of my own personal story as well as my professional experience over the last twenty years helping hundreds of clients, men and women alike, look and feel their best and achieve optimal health, and educating them on what it really takes to lose body fat and keep it off.

As I began hiking one day, I quietly said to myself, "God, if you want me to write another book, please give me a sign. During this hike, if I see a butterfly, that will be my sign that I should move forward with my desire to share my knowledge in another book." At the very end of my hike, not only one, but three beautiful yellow butterflies appeared. It was awesome…magical. I got chills. Therefore, it is with pure pleasure, passion and desire to empower you and inspire you on your journey to achieve lasting fat loss success that I present to you my second book, *Fat Loss Revolution.* Thank you, God!

*From my heart* ♥

*Always with love,*

*Paula Owens*

## INTRODUCTION

## FOCUS ON HEALTH FIRST AND FAT LOSS WILL HAPPEN

F*at Loss Revolution* is NOT a book about the next best celebrity diet, nor is it about calories in versus calories out, exercising more and eating less. The *Fat Loss Revolution* is not a quick fix program where you'll lose weight and eventually regain it all back plus some extra. The *Fat Loss Revolution* is a book about a process to strategically achieve your permanent fat loss goals forever.

If you've been struggling and failing time and time again to lose weight by exercising more and eating less, the *Fat Loss Revolution* is your answer. You probably feel discouraged, disheartened or frustrated. Please release these feelings from your mind, body and soul altogether. Fat loss resistance is not your fault. Sustainable and healthy fat loss entails so much more than starvation dieting and excessive exercise. Underlying imbalances can inhibit any effort to lose body fat. In fact, poor sleep habits, hormonal fluctuations, your emotional state, chemical imbalances in the brain, environmental toxins and stress levels can all affect your ability to lose fat.

The *Fat Loss Revolution* will educate and inform you with nutritional and lifestyle know-how to help you lose body fat permanently and in a healthy manner. In *Fat Loss Revolution* you will find my secrets to attain optimal health and permanent fat loss that have worked time and time again, not only for myself personally, but for thousands of men and women.

The *Fat Loss Revolution* is a process – a recipe for long-lasting success – a lifestyle, not a quick fix. My intention is to empower you to reach your goals by providing enlightening information that you can incorporate into your daily routines so it becomes part of your everyday life. The end result will be a "hot 'n healthy body" no matter what your age. In just 12 weeks, you will look and feel better than you ever have if you follow the principles laid out in the *Fat Loss Revolution.*

Two thirds of Americans are now medically classified as overweight or obese. According to a survey published in the July 2011 issue of *Life Extension,* 30 percent of overweight individuals mistakenly believe they are at a healthy weight, and 70 percent of obese individuals think they're simply overweight. This excess weight is costing our nation approximately $93 billion annually in medical bills!

A study by the Organization for Economic Cooperation and Development predicts that by 2020, nearly 75 percent of the American population will be overweight or obese. What does this mean? It means that by 2020, more than half of all Americans are at risk of developing pre-diabetic conditions or suffering from type 2 diabetes. Sadly, it also means that as a nation of excess in every aspect, our health is deteriorating.

Visit any mall, school or amusement park, and you will witness the devastation of expanding waistlines. Why are waistlines expanding so rapidly? In part, the obesity epidemic is attributed to changes in our environment, including the prevalence of energy-dense food, several lifestyle factors and behaviors such as alcohol intake, television watching and sleep deprivation, which encourage excessive eating.

People are eating massive portions void of nutrients and filled with too many carbohydrates that end up spiking insulin and causing excess fat gain. In *Chapter 2,* you will discover why and how this happens. For now, let's just suffice it to say that excess can lead to a mess.

The *Fat Loss Revolution* breaks the traditional approach to losing weight. This book will provide you with all of the important elements you need to get healthy, prevent disease, change your body, transform your life and lose body fat in just 12 weeks – at any age.

# It Starts With Choices

Over the next 12 weeks, choose to keep an open mind. Consciously set aside what you think you know about fat loss and allow the information provided in the *Fat Loss Revolution* to govern your choices. Focus your energy on the variety of lifestyle adjustments you will be informed about. My promise to you is that if you do this, you will achieve the results you are looking for long-term.

Your personal transformation begins with making the choice to change your mindset and vision for your life. After that, other vital areas where healthier choices must be made will be discussed. These areas include choosing activities and nutrition that will balance your hormones, developing better sleep patterns, improving digestion and absorption of nutrients, melting unwanted body fat and making better choices in all areas of your life. All of these topics and more are an integral part of losing body fat.

As you learn and incorporate the information provided in the *Fat Loss Revolution* into your life, you will see how your choices influence and lead you to living a fuller, healthier, happier life.

The information in the *Fat Loss Revolution* will provide you with answers and multiple options so you can strategize and prioritize your journey to optimal health and wellness.

As you follow the recommendations in the *Fat Loss Revolution,* you will look and feel better, sleep sounder, experience flatter abs and reduce your body fat in just 12 weeks.

One of my favorite quotes is from world-renowned Olympic strength coach Charles Poliquin: *"No one ever ate anything by accident."* That being said, the next choice to make is deciding that there will be no more excuses – dietary or otherwise.

Now is the time to create balance in your life, taking control and responsibility for any unhealthy habits and choices in the past that have contributed to excess body fat and adverse health conditions.

It is with kindness and compassion for you and your success that I say, "Own the choices you have made." Address any attitudes that have led to the behaviors and underlying patterns of poor choices made in the past. Be completely honest and then let it go and resolve to proceed with your personal *Fat Loss Revolution*. Making this investment pays substantial dividends. Shifting your mindset will allow you to make better choices effortlessly. Remember that growth is incremental. Even the longest journey begins with one small step. Focus your thoughts toward becoming healthy. Doing so will result in fat loss that will happen naturally.

You are worth every bit of the time, energy and effort it takes to accomplish your personal transformation. Make a choice and commitment right now. Invest in yourself.

**Let's get this *Fat Loss Revolution* started!**

# 12 Weeks to a Hot 'N Healthy Body at Any Age

Losing fat takes more than a desire. It takes commitment, a determined mindset, realistic goals, consistency, balanced hormones and a well-designed lifestyle plan that is practiced and followed continually so that it becomes a lifestyle. Whether your goal is to lose body fat, stabilize your blood sugar and prevent the risk of diabetes, or look and feel your best ever, the principles found in the *Fat Loss Revolution* will work for a lifetime.

Any results-oriented program that is not a quick-fix requires at least 12 weeks of faithful participation, consistency and compliance to experience real results.

Going back to what was discussed about mindset – be aware that when any area of your life is out of balance, choices can be negatively affected. Experiencing varying degrees of worry, stress, anxiety and frustration also affect your ability to make healthier choices and can inhibit fat loss.

Most people look at their diet or exercise habits as the perfect twosome to achieve fat loss. Yes, both diet and exercise are extremely important aspects in the fat loss equation. However, many other factors and principles cannot be overlooked and must be part of the overall fat loss dynamic.

Each one of us is a unique human being. The perfect solution that worked for your sister, your friend or your trainer may not work for you. Your genetic makeup can cause you to metabolize fat differently than your friend even though you both followed the exact same program. The information in the *Fat Loss Revolution* will powerfully influence your genetic propensity.

> *Successful fat loss requires thinking and acting outside the conventional weight loss box.*

# *Fat Loss Revolution* Principles

Below are the *Fat Loss Revolution* principles to achieve permanent fat loss. Many of these topics are often overlooked when it comes to losing body fat and more importantly, keeping it off.

* Balancing hormones
* Reducing and preventing inflammation
* An efficient and healthy functioning metabolism

* Eliminating intolerant foods, chemicals, addictive foods
* Consuming an unrestrictive diet of wholesome, organic foods
* Periodic detoxification

* A smart, sensible, effective exercise program
* Optimal digestion
* Quality relationships
* Recognition that each person responds differently

* Restful sleep
* Stress management
* Addressing nutritional deficiencies
* Positive thinking and emotional well-being

# CHAPTER 1

## WEIGHT LOSS VS. FAT LOSS FOR A HOT 'N HEALTHY BODY

First and foremost, what many people neglect to take into consideration is the major difference between weight loss and fat loss.

When you're obsessed with weighing yourself on the scale, you're solely focused on *"weight loss."* An individual's weight can fluctuate during the day, especially when you factor in fluid retention, sodium intake and muscle weight. The scale is not an accurate method of tracking *"fat loss."* Just because the number on the scale is going down does not mean you are losing fat. You may be losing water weight and muscle. Losing muscle is not ideal because muscle tissue is metabolically active and helps burn body fat.

Muscle tissue is much denser than fat tissue and muscle takes up less space in the body. When you workout consistently and intelligently, your lean muscle tissue increases and your body fat decreases. This is why the scale is not your best tool for monitoring fat loss. Two individuals can have the same exact body weight and height, but have completely different body compositions and body dimensions. On the other hand, two individuals can have an equal body fat percentage, but the leaner person will weigh more on the scale due to the higher density/weight of lean muscle tissue.

In contrast, fat loss is about focusing your energy and efforts toward building and maintaining lean muscle tissue.

> *Genuinely embrace that there is a difference between short-term weight loss and long-term fat loss.*

The *Fat Loss Revolution* program is designed so you lose body fat exclusively, preserve lean muscle tissue and minimize muscle loss in order to achieve a body that is lean, fit and healthy – inside and out.

Remember, fat loss is NOT about counting calories, starvation diets, measuring food, stepping on the scale every day, willpower or excessive amounts of exercise. Instead, fat loss is about building and keeping muscle, your metabolically active tissue; choosing higher quality, nutrient-dense foods; intelligent exercise; balanced hormones; and factoring in all the other lifestyle aspects (sleep, stress, etc.) of fat loss that are often overlooked.

Did you know that as we age, a cause and a symptom of the aging process is sarcopenia? Sarcopenia simply means the degenerative loss of skeletal muscle mass and strength associated with aging. Sarcopenia also leads to an overall weakness and a decline in metabolic rate due to less muscle mass. With a lower metabolic rate, losing body fat becomes more challenging. The good news is that implementing the methods and principles set forth in the *Fat Loss Revolution* will help you put an end to this vicious cycle. Instead, you will gain more muscle so you can burn more calories and lose any unwanted body fat.

> Bottom line – the more lean muscle mass you have, the higher your metabolic rate and the longer you will live.

# Monitor Body Composition for Fat Loss

Although hydrostatic or underwater weighing is considered an accurate method of determining body composition (body fat to lean mass), it is not the most practical mode of testing. Another common method to assess body composition is bioimpedance; however the margin of error can be quite drastic depending upon hydration status, food in the stomach or during menstruation thereby giving an unreliable and false reading.

My personal recommendation for accurately assessing fat loss is measuring body composition with skinfold calipers, not stepping on a scale. Ideally, it is best to take measurements at the same time of the day on a bi-weekly basis. A realistic goal for long-term fat loss is 0.5 percent fat loss each week, which is equivalent to one to two pounds of fat loss per week.

Calculating body composition with skinfold calipers is by far a superior gauge for assessing fat loss as compared to using the body mass index (BMI). My preferred method for assessing fat loss is the Poliquin™ BioSignature Modulation.

BioSignature Modulation is a 12-site body fat composition testing protocol developed by world-renowned Olympic Strength Coach Charles Poliquin. The 12 sites tested reveal your personal hormone profile and detect hormonal imbalances responsible for where and how much body fat you store.

BioSignature Modulation, when performed correctly by a skilled and qualified BioSignature Modulation practitioner using Harpenden skinfold calipers, yields amazing results over time because it goes beyond standard body fat testing and provides you with a personalized blueprint for faster fat loss. For this reason, Poliquin™ BioSignature Modulation is being embraced by many of the top functional medicine practitioners in the United States.

For more information, go to PaulaOwens.com/programs.html.

## Healthy body fat percentages

According to the American College of Sports Medicine essential fat is the minimal amount of fat necessary for normal physiological function. Essential fat values for males are typically considered to be 3 percent and 12 percent for women. Fat above the minimal amount is referred to as nonessential fat. It is generally accepted that a range of 10-18 percent for men and 20-25 percent for women is considered satisfactory and healthy limits. For a leaner, more athletic-looking physique, men can aim for 7-11 percent and women can aim for 15-22 percent without compromising health.

A body composition within the recommended range suggests less risk of developing obesity-related diseases such as diabetes, high blood pressure, and even some cancers. In addition, although there are risks when body composition is too high, there are also risks when body composition is too low. Body fat levels below the minimal recommended levels of essential fat, negatively affect the delivery of vitamins to the organs, the ability of the reproductive system to function, and overall well-being.

## Other methods to track fat loss success vs. the scale

### Circumference measurements

On Saturday or Sunday morning, take your circumference measurements with a tape measure and record them in your journal. Measure weekly on the same day of the week.

**Above chest** – Place a tape measure around your chest directly under your armpits. Lower your arms. Read and record the measurement.

**Chest** – Position the tape measure around your chest over the nipple area. Read and record the measurement.

**Waist** – To find your waist, lean to the left and locate the area halfway between your hip bone and your bottom rib. Stand upright and place the measuring tape around your waist. Read and record your measurement.

**Navel** – Place the tape measure around your body at the location of your bellybutton. Read and record your measurement.

**Hips** – Stand sideways with feet together, looking in a mirror, and locate the roundest area of your glutes (buttocks). Place the tape measure at this point around your hips. Read and record your measurement.

**Thighs** – Stand with your legs and feet together. Place the tape measure around the top of both legs directly underneath your glutes. Read and record your measurement.

## Photos

You've heard that pictures don't lie. As you embark on your *Fat Loss Revolution* journey, take photos as soon as possible so you can see your visual transformation.

Every week have someone take photos of your body as you stand facing the front, the side, and the rear. Photos should be taken at the same time of day, and on the same day each week. Make sure both you and the photographer stand in the same place at the same distance from each other when taking the photos.

Men should wear black shorts. Women should wear a black sports bra and black shorts. Post your photos where you can see them often in your house or office.

## Next size down: Fit-into-my-jeans test

How your clothes fit, especially your blue jeans, is a great way to determine if you're on track with your *Fat Loss Revolution* transformation. Maybe you have a favorite pair of jeans that you struggle to squeeze into, or a favorite dress that no longer fits because it's just a bit too tight. Perhaps you currently wear a size 14 and you'd love to wear a size 6.

How your clothes fit can be used as an alternative method to track your fat loss progress throughout the next 12 weeks. One way to do this is to find a specific pair of jeans that you're trying to fit into. Once a week, on the same day of the week, first thing in the morning, try on your jeans for the "fit-into-my-jeans" test. For instance, when you start the fit into my jeans test, let's say that you can barely get your jeans past your knees. Each week as you try on your jeans, notice how your jeans fit. If your jeans couldn't get past your knees, and this week they do, you are moving in the right direction and making progress!

# CHAPTER 2

## HEALTHY HORMONES FOR A HOT 'N HEALTHY BODY

Hormones are powerful chemical messengers that communicate and transport information to your cells and organs. It only takes a small amount of a hormone to cause major changes in cells or your whole body. Hormones affect many different bodily processes, including reproduction, sleep, mood, detoxification, appetite, digestion, libido and metabolism.

## What do hormones have to do with fat loss?

The body is comprised of many systems that are interconnected: the endocrine, nervous, respiratory, immune, digestive, musculoskeletal, cardiovascular, urinary, integumentary and reproductive systems. No system of the body works in isolation. With that being said, hormones do not act independently. All hormones work together to create balance and homeostasis, and to enhance utilization of stored body fat. When one hormone is disrupted, it influences all of the other hormones. Attention to hormonal balance *must* be factored in when it comes to lowering body fat composition.

Here's a common scenario: You are eating a healthy diet, consistent with a smart exercise program, and still struggling to lose body fat. How frustrating! What's going on here? Hormone imbalances!

Hormonal imbalances can caused by excessive stress, poor digestion, insulin resistance, unknown food sensitivities, a toxic or congested liver, PMS and peri-menopause, hidden inflammation, lack of sleep or nutrient deficiencies. Minor hormonal imbalances can cause symptoms ranging from an inability to lose weight to fatigue to uncontrollable sugar, carbohydrate or alcohol cravings.

There are many factors that affect hormonal status and how your body burns and stores fat, including the types of food you eat and the beverages you drink, along with your sleep patterns, type of exercise you engage in, stress levels, nutrient status, and deficiencies. These all influence the balance or imbalance of your hormones.

Let's discuss the hormones that inhibit fat loss and tend to cause the majority of health problems.

## Insulin

Insulin is a major hormone that regulates blood sugar levels and has many actions within the body. It is your primary regulator of fat metabolism and it is the most important hormone when it comes to fat loss. One of the functions of insulin is fat storage. Insulin increases fat production. It is the number one hormone you have control over. How? By what you choose to eat!

The role of insulin in fat loss is to remove excess glucose from the blood stream and store it in the liver and muscles as glycogen, or into adipose (fat) tissue as triglycerides. If you want to win the war on fat loss, one of your primary goals should be to create an environment where you body is sensitive to insulin so any sugars you consume deposit into the muscle and liver cells, not your fat cells.

Different foods you choose to eat create different hormonal (insulin) responses in the body. For example, eating vegetables with a protein has an insignificant and favorable effect on blood sugar and will keep your body sensitive to insulin. On the other hand, snacking on gummy bears, a bagel, fruit juice or a frozen yogurt with cookie crumbles will send your insulin levels through the roof. Sugary treats and excess carbohydrates are the perfect fuel source if you want to add fat around your midsection and create that puffy muffin-top look.

> *The quality and quantity of carbohydrates you eat have a direct influence on your body fat levels.*

When you eat a meal high in carbohydrates, they are broken down into glucose (sugar). Insulin levels in the blood are correlated to the amount of carbohydrates and sugar you consume.

Carbohydrates are sugars. Even agave, although natural, is still a sugar. It has an effect similar to high-fructose corn syrup, triggering insulin secretion, which signals your body to accumulate fat.

When you consume processed carbohydrates, grains and sugar, your body senses the glucose and releases insulin from the pancreas to clear the sugars from the bloodstream. Insulin transports glucose into your cells, with the primary destination for glucose being your fat cells. Therefore, to turn your insulin profile around to favor insulin sensitivity, limit consumption of refined carbohydrates, grains and sugars and you'll be leaner. On the other hand, the higher your intake of carbohydrates, grains and sugar, the more fat you'll store.

Rapid spikes in blood sugar are not favorable for fat loss. High insulin levels suppress two vital fat-releasing hormones – glucagon and growth hormones – which are responsible for burning fat and muscle development. Blood sugar fluctuations and insulin spikes create an environment to gain fat. And if that isn't bad enough, insulin spikes cause muscle loss, and over time high levels of insulin can induce major long-term damage to your body.

Balanced insulin levels are crucial not only for losing body fat, but also for reducing mid-section belly fat that tends to occur during menopause or andropause. Stabilizing insulin is vital to prevent diabetes, anxiety and depression, heart disease, dementia, stroke and cancer.

**Insulin resistance and pre-diabetes** are both indications that the cell has lost its responsiveness on the insulin receptor site – particularly liver, muscle and fat cells, with the liver losing sensitivity first, followed by muscle, then fat cells.

The blood sugar and insulin roller coaster will damage your ability to use insulin properly, causing excess insulin, thereby storing more body fat. Over time, the pancreas gives up, leading to type 2 diabetes.

Insulin resistance is the number one primary factor of nearly every chronic disease and health condition, including weight gain. Individuals who are insulin-resistant tend to carry excess fat around their mid-sections.

This excess belly fat is a sign that you are becoming increasingly insulin resistant. It is well-established that midsection fat accumulation significantly increases risk of degenerative disease and related health problems.

**What causes insulin resistance?**
* A diet heavy in grains, sugar and carbohydrates
* A sedentary lifestyle
* Bisphenol–A and Bisphenol–S (BPA and BPS) exposure
* Excess omega-6 fatty acids in relationship to omega-3 fatty acids
* Inflammation
* Low protein intake
* Processed, packaged and fatty foods
* Consumption of high-fructose corn syrup
* Prolonged, restricted dieting
* Skipping meals, especially breakfast
* Stress, adrenal fatigue, altered hormones (elevated cortisol)

Evidence published in the September 2005 issue of the *International Journal of Obesity* supports Dr. Robert Lustig's theory of a direct connection between elevated insulin levels and the relationship to weight gain and obesity. Dr. Lustig is the professor of Clinical Pediatrics at UCSF Center for Obesity, and specializes in addressing the role hormones play in weight and behavior.

For instance, when you eat a bagel or a piece of bread, it is quickly digested and turned into glucose. Glucose levels rise and trigger additional insulin secretion to keep up with the surge of glucose in the blood.

Those who crave carbohydrates are often serotonin deficient because the release of insulin has the effect of increasing brain levels of serotonin.

Refined carbohydrates including bagels, bread, pasta, pretzels, breakfast cereals and most other processed foods break down rapidly into sugar, triggering a rise in insulin levels, which in turn causes unwanted fat storage as well as insulin resistance if these food choices continue long-term.

> *Carbohydrates drive insulin.*
> *Insulin drives fat storage.*

Insulin resistance is a progressive problem that continually gets worse over time. Insulin resistance significantly increases your risk for breast cancer, stroke, cholesterol irregularities, dementia, high blood pressure, heart disease, osteoporosis, and other diseases and medical problems.

In order to accurately determine if you're pre-diabetic or insulin-resistant, have your blood sugar, insulin and hemoglobin A1C levels measured. Be sure to fast 10 to 12 hours prior to testing for accuracy.

**Insulin sensitivity** is your body's ability to use insulin properly to regulate the amount of glucose in the bloodstream. To encourage greater fat loss, you want to create an environment in which you're sensitive to insulin. When you're sensitive to insulin, you will be less likely to become a fat-storing machine because your body will transport glucose into the muscles and not the fat cells.

### *Revolution Solutions* to increase insulin sensitivity

* Reduce your intake of sugars, grains, refined carbohydrates and all processed, packaged and junk foods and avoid all products with high-fructose corn syrup.

* Limit fructose and keep consumption of fruit to one to two servings daily. Excessive fructose consumption, even from fruit, will inhibit your fat loss efforts. Choose fruits such as berries, which are high in fiber, full of nutrients and have a lower glycemic load. The polyphenols in berries inhibit the formation of new fat cells and help to break down stored fat.

* Strength train with weights, which is far superior to steady state aerobic-style exercise (see *Chapter 11*) for increasing insulin sensitivity.

* Increase intake of organic protein. An article published in the *Nutrition Journal* concluded that a low-carb, high-protein diet is better than a low-fat diet to reduce insulin levels and improve insulin sensitivity.

* Drink organic green tea, white tea and organic coffee.

* Get seven to nine hours of sleep. Lack of sleep creates hormonal disruption by reducing insulin sensitivity, increasing cortisol and decreasing growth hormone.

* Balance the ratio of omega-3 fatty acids to omega-6 fatty acids. Eliminate intake of trans-fatty acids, hydrogenated and partially hydrogenated oils and all vegetable oils including canola, safflower, corn and soy. Increase consumption of wild-caught fish or pharmaceutical-grade, molecularly-distilled liquid fish oil or capsules.

* Increase insulin sensitivity with zinc, magnesium, grapeseed extract, vitamin D, resveratrol, probiotics, chromium, curcumin, alpha lipoic acid (R-ALA) and carnitine.

Longevity studies of all creatures, from worms and yeasts to humans, show that the lower the levels of insulin are over the course of one's life, the longer the life will be. The *Fat Loss Revolution* eating plan, exercise programs and lifestyle principles encourage an environment that will increase insulin sensitivity.

## Thyroid

Your thyroid is the master gland of your metabolism, the rate at which you burn fat. It is your body's internal thermostat, regulating your temperature by secreting two hormones, T3 and T4, which control your ability to burn calories and use energy. The thyroid controls your weight, body temperature, heart rate, energy levels, menstrual regularity and muscle strength. If your thyroid is low by one percent, it affects your metabolism by six percent, meaning that if your thyroid is low by 10 percent, your metabolism will be slowed by 60 percent.

Approximately 27 million Americans experience an underactive thyroid, and less than 25 percent of those with an underactive thyroid have been diagnosed properly and treated.

**Hypothyroid symptoms** include, but are not limited to:
* Weight gain despite a healthy diet and a smart exercise program
* Low energy levels
* Dry skin and hair loss
* Brain fog
* Loss of the outer third portion of the eyebrows
* Depression
* Low body temperature
* Morning headaches that wear off as the day progresses
* Overly sensitive to cold weather
* Chronic digestive problems

Some early symptoms of hypothyroid are mistaken for fatigue, anxiety or aging. Sugar intolerance, menopause and depression all have similarities to thyroid disorders. Untreated hypothyroidism dramatically increases your risk of serious health concerns and degenerative diseases.

## Stress and thyroid function

Thyroid hormones are affected by stress. Adrenaline, noradrenaline and cortisol, hormones released under stressful conditions by the adrenal glands, interfere with the body's ability to convert T4 into T3. When T3 levels decrease, the body produces even more adrenaline and cortisol to help speed up metabolism, which further inhibits the conversion of T4 to T3.

When your adrenal glands are overworked, your body converts progesterone into adrenal hormones, resulting in depleted progesterone levels. When progesterone lowers due to the conversion into stress hormones, the thyroid comes to the rescue to remove stress from the body. If the adrenals are exhausted, the thyroid steps in to maintain sufficient production of adrenal hormones.

The endocrine system is unable to deal with this process long-term. Eventually, the thyroid decreases hormone production to conserve energy. Initially, there may be thyroid and the adrenal dysfunction, but eventually it is usually the thyroid that suffers. This is why healthy functioning adrenals must be factored in when thyroid hormones are out of range.

## Determine the cause of a sluggish thyroid

Pre-disposing factors and thyroid disruptors include:

*   Adrenal insufficiency. Healthy functioning adrenals must *always* be factored in when dealing with thyroid imbalances.

*   Celiac disease and gluten intolerance. It is especially important that people with hypothyroid or thyroid autoimmune diseases to avoid gluten and millet.

*   Prolonged chemical exposure (FD&C red dye #3, parabens, pesticides, phthalates, perchlorates, PCBs, etc.)

*   Diets high in sugar, carbohydrates and grains, specifically wheat

*   Estrogen dominance and progesterone insufficiency

*   Fatty acid deficiency or protein insufficiency

*   Excess exposure to:
    *   fluoride (toothpaste, unfiltered water, some teas, processed foods, conventional meat and dairy). Fluoride displaces iodine in the thyroid.
    *   bromine (pools, hot tubs, cereals, pasta, commercially baked breads; also found in mattresses, computers, carpet, furniture and electronic gadgets; also a fire retardant)
    *   chlorine (unfiltered water, toothpaste, some brands of tea, processed foods and prescription drugs)

*   Insulin resistance

*   Liver congestion and gallbladder dysfunction

*   Nutritional deficiencies (zinc, iodine, selenium, vitamin A, D and B vitamins). The thyroid and the adrenals need vitamin A to work efficiently.

* Digestive dysfunction and absorption issues

* Gut flora imbalances

* Food sensitivities that increase inflammation (food sensitivities are very common in those with hypothyroidism)

* Soy isoflavones (should be eliminated)

* Rule out viruses and heavy metal body burdens (common in individuals with hypothyroidism)

## Suggested thyroid tests

**At-home thyroid self-test.** Before going to bed, set a glass basal thermometer on your nightstand. The moment you wake up, place the thermometer under your left armpit for 10 minutes. (This would be the perfect time to set your intention – a plan, goal, prayer or desire – for the day). Monitor your temperature for five consecutive days. Total the number, then divide by five for an average temperature.

A morning temperature consistently less than 97.8°F *may* suggest hypothyroidism, whereas temperatures consistently less than 97.3°F are highly probable of low thyroid function.

If there is suspicion based on the results of the at-home self-test, or continued symptoms of a sluggish thyroid are present, follow through with lab testing.

To accurately determine and diagnose thyroid function, obtain a comprehensive, clinical evaluation conducted by a qualified health practitioner. Measuring different hormones in the blood can determine if the thyroid gland is working properly; however, subjective indicators should not be overlooked.

Traditional labs often miss the mark when it comes to assessing thyroid hormones. If your doctor is only testing TSH (thyroid stimulating hormone) to determine thyroid function, it may be time to find a new doctor. For a more accurate diagnosis, there are eight recommended lab tests as listed here:

**Lab testing for thyroid function**

**Thyroid Stimulating Hormone (TSH).** Beware of the so-called "normal" ranges: most are simply dead wrong. The ideal level for TSH is between 1 and 1.5 mIU/L.

**T4 Panel**
Free T4 – normal level of free T4 is between 0.9 and 1.8 ng/dl
T4 Thyroxine – optimal levels are 8-12.5
Free Thyroxine Index – optimal levels are 1.5-5

**T3 Panel**
Free T3 – optimal ranges are 1.8-5.4
T3 Uptake – optimal levels are 27-37
T3 Total – optimal ranges are 72-170
Reverse T3

**Thyroid Peroxidase Antibody**. Optimal ranges are 0-19

**TPO-Ab.** Optimal range is <35

**Adrenal Function**
DHEA and DHEA-S
Adrenal Stress Index (ASI)

**Candida and Heavy Metal Body Burdens.** Both Candida and heavy metal toxicity are very common in those with hypothyroidism.

**Homocysteine.** Clinical research has shown that homocystinuria is found with many cases of primary and secondary thyroid hypo-function.

### *Revolution Solutions* for an underactive thyroid

The good news is that once you have assessed and confirmed that your thyroid is sluggish, there are healing strategies to help correct and balance your thyroid.

Nutritional support for a sluggish thyroid will be specific to each individual and may include:

* Iodine/iodide, a critical building block (Note: Peer review literature indicates that iodine should be restricted in those with increased thyroid antibodies.)
* Selenium, especially for autoimmune thyroid conditions
* L-tyrosine, an amino acid used by the thyroid gland. It works with iodine to activate T3 and T4.
* Digestzymes to support digestion and absorption of nutrients
* Adrenal support
* Vitamins D and A
* Omega-3 fatty acids
* Sea vegetables (kelp, dulsi, nori, wakame), seafood (wild salmon, oysters, sardines, shrimp), sesame seeds, iodized sea salt

EPA and DHA, the omega-3 fatty acids in fish oil, have been found to help boost thyroid hormones within the liver cells to burn fat. Several studies, including a study published in the *Journal of Lipids,* have shown that those who consumed a diet higher in omega-3 fats had significantly less accumulation of body fat.

## Cortisol

Cortisol is a hormone produced by the adrenal glands. Besides assisting in hormone production, cortisol is produced in response to stress, keeps your blood sugar stable, suppresses the immune system, and aids in fat, carbohydrate and protein metabolism. Adrenaline (epinephrine), noradrenaline (norepinephrine) and cortisol are referred to as the "fight-or-flight" hormones. The brain has the ability to selectively activate the fight, flight or defeat response.

When you experience extended periods of stress and anxiety, you may experience depression or feelings of surrender or giving up, which also cause your adrenal glands to release cortisol. As a result of the fight-or-flight stress responses, the heart beats faster and harder. The pupils of the eyes dilate, the release of natural pain inhibitors is stimulated and more glucose and fats are released into the blood. According to the University of Mexico, the defeat response can lead to increased lipogenesis (fat creation), visceral obesity (deep abdominal fat), bone and muscle atrophy, accelerated aging and suppression of the immune system.

As we age, the adrenal glands also become the control center for many hormones, including cortisol, adrenaline, DHEA, progesterone, aldosterone, estrogen and testosterone. As estrogen and progesterone levels fluctuate during mid-life, balanced cortisol and insulin are of utmost importance to prevent the excess belly fat that tends to occur during menopause. In essence, your adrenal glands become your back-up pharmacy. It is especially important that you have healthy functioning adrenals (cortisol) and balanced blood sugar (insulin) entering into menopause or andropause because the adrenal glands produce 40 percent of your sex hormones before menopause or andropause and 90 ninety percent after menopause or andropause. Consequently, the stronger the adrenals, the easier your shift into menopause or andropause will be.

Cortisol is produced and rises in response to stressors such as pain and inflammation, glycemic control and psychological overload. Fasting for long periods of time, food intake, over-exercising, awakening and psychosocial stressors all cause the body to release cortisol.

Higher levels of cortisol boost your energy, which is why you want high cortisol in the morning and not at night. Those experiencing adrenal fatigue have elevated levels of cortisol at the wrong time of the day, meaning they are experiencing a surge of energy after 6:00 p.m. instead of during the earlier part of the day when cortisol should be at its highest.

Cortisol directly affects fat storage and weight gain in overly stressed individuals because it indirectly influences appetite and cravings for sugar, carbs and fat by regulating other chemicals that are released during stress. Although the stress pathways work together, they each can uniquely affect the function of various bodily processes.

Many women taking birth control pills tend to experience higher levels of cortisol. A study presented at the 122nd Annual Meeting of the American Physiological Society revealed that concentrations of anabolic hormones (hormones that promote tissue and muscle synthesis) were lower in women taking oral contraceptives, and cortisol was elevated.

Resting and digesting are considered to be parasympathetic states and most natural for the body. Fast-paced lifestyles force the sympathetic nervous system (the opposite of parasympathetic) into overdrive, wreaking havoc on the adrenal glands. The adrenal glands become overstimulated from lack of sleep, addiction to stimulants, operating on overdrive 24-7, accumulative stress, over-exercising (especially aerobic/cardio) and eating poor quality foods. All of these create biochemical imbalances that inhibit your ability to lose body fat.

Hormones such as cortisol and thyroid are anabolic (building up) at low levels and catabolic (breaking down) at rising and high levels. Anabolic function favors the synthesis of hormones, enzymes and peptides. Catabolic function activates glycolysis (or breakdown of glycogen, which releases glucose) and blocks uptake of glucose by peripheral tissues, creating a hyperglycemic state.

High cortisol levels can disrupt sleep, mood, metabolism, mental focus and eating habits. When cortisol levels are chronically high, muscle is lost and fat is gained, particularly in the abdominal region, in both men and women. Elevated levels of cortisol are associated with overeating and craving high-calorie fatty and sugary foods. Over time, elevated levels of cortisol relocate fat from the circulation and storage depots to the deep internal abdominal area, increasing visceral fat (the fat surrounding the organs).

Excess cortisol is also directly associated with subcutaneous fat accumulation, the fat directly under your skin that you can pinch or grab. Depleted levels of cortisol can occur from chronic stress causing you to feel exhausted, fatigued and unmotivated, resulting in adrenal exhaustion.

It has been proven that people with diseases associated with extreme exposure to cortisol, such as severe recurrent depression and Cushing's disease, also have excessive amounts of visceral fat. In addition, elevated cortisol has been linked to hypertension (high blood pressure), hyperlipidemia (elevated lipids), hyperglycemia (elevated glucose) and an increased risk of depression.

Now that it has been established that high cortisol levels are detrimental to health and negate fat loss efforts, how does an individual lower their cortisol to a normal, healthy level?

* Control cortisol with the *Fat Loss Revolution* eating plan, which includes plenty of organic protein and non-starchy vegetables.
* Eliminate foods your body is sensitive to (see *Chapter 5*).
* Rule out pathogenic gut infections. Common culprits include yeast or fungal overgrowth otherwise known as Candida, H. pylori, C. difficile and parasites.
* Optimize gut function (see *Chapter 6*).
* Adopt the simple habit of drinking more water to prevent dehydration, which helps to lower cortisol.
* Exercise. Although exercise elevates cortisol, the appropriate type and amount of exercise will not chronically elevate cortisol (see *Chapter 11*).
* Develop a healthier lifestyle that includes getting enough sleep and relaxation; stress-reducing activities such as meditation, yoga, leisure walks and deep breathing techniques; and being outdoors in nature.

*Slow, deep, belly breathing helps reduce the stress response and lower cortisol levels. Take a deep breath in through your nose, inhale to a count of four, hold it for two seconds, and exhale the air through your mouth as you meditate on your favorite mantra. Pause for one second and repeat this at least eight cycles to reset your stress response.*

The best way to determine your cortisol level is with a saliva test called the Adrenal Stress Index (ASI). The ASI test is reliable and non-invasive, and can help you evaluate whether your stress levels are cause for concern. This test evaluates how well the adrenal glands function by tracking their 24-hour circadian rhythm. Saliva samples are taken four times/day for one day to determine your basic cortisol rhythm.

**Nutritional support** to help lower cortisol levels is specific to each individual and may include, but is not limited to:

* Magnesium
* Phosphatadylserine
* RLC Labs – Adrenal Support
* Biotics Research – ABD5 Plus
* Omega-3 fatty acids
* Vitamin C
* Rhodiola
* Probiotics

### Remember these facts:

*In order to balance your cortisol levels, you must first stabilize your blood sugar.*

*If your adrenals are exhausted, it will be difficult to balance your other hormones. Hormones do not act independently.*

*A healthy functioning digestive system is required to support and nourish your adrenals (see Chapter 6).*

# Estrogen

Estrogen dominance is an unhealthy condition in which the body has accumulated an overabundance of estrogen. This is a very common and increasingly serious problem today that affects not only men and women, but also our youth.

Estrogen dominance generally occurs when there is an imbalance between estrogen and progesterone. As men approach their 40s, testosterone levels decline and often much of their remaining testosterone converts to estrogen, a process known as aromatization. Men may experience prostate problems, weight gain, hair loss, atherosclerosis, gynecomastia (male breast development), lowered libido and impotency.

Estrogen dominance in women tends to appear in their 30s and 40s, although younger women can suffer from estrogen dominance. As women approach menopause, progesterone levels fluctuate as the ratio of estrogen to progesterone is high. Symptoms women may experience include breast tenderness, heavy menses, cellulite and an increased risk of fibroids, endometriosis, breast cancer, stroke and heart disease. In women, estrogen overload increases fat storage and cellulite in the lower body, whereas men tend to experience fat storage in their chest area (breast tissue).

When excess estrogen accumulates in the liver, symptoms such as depression, weight gain, constipation, cellulite, cyclical headaches and migraines, mood swings, fluid retention and low libido can be experienced as well as many other symptoms. According to Harvard physician John R. Lee., M.D, "Anything that impairs liver function or ties up the detoxifying function will result in excess estrogen levels."

Estrogen dominance can also develop as a result of the aging process, a poor diet, hormone dysfunction, chronic stress, overusing alcohol, excess inflammation, plant estrogens (soy), prescription drug use, birth control pills, hormone replacement therapy (HRT), obesity, environmental factors and liver congestion. Quite a lengthy list!

Those with estrogen dominance have increased alpha andregenic receptors – *fat storage* receptors that block the release of fat. Beta andregenic receptors are *fat burning* receptors that increase the release of fat.

According to research by Braun and Horton in 2001, abdominal adipocytes are more sensitive to beta receptor stimulation than hip and thigh adipocytes in both men and women. Women tend to have more alpha receptors in their lower body, which has a direct influence on estrogen because fat is attracted to estrogen. Fat is metabolically active tissue that is also capable of producing estrogen. This is one of the reasons women experience cellulite and have a harder time losing body fat from their hips, buttocks and thighs.

Endocrine-disrupting chemicals (EDCs) are known as obesogens. Obesogens mimic or alter the effects of hormones in the body and often target the estrogen receptors. Obesogens inappropriately alter lipid homeostasis and fat storage, change metabolic set points, disrupt energy balance or modify the regulation of appetite and satiety to promote fat accumulation and obesity (see *Chapter 7*).

Xenoestrogens, a type of obesogen, are environmental, man-made chemicals with a chemical structure similar to estrogen that accumulate in fatty human tissue. The longer these foreign substances stay in your body the more opportunity they have to do damage. Research has shown that xenoestrogens can interfere with the body's signaling pathways by binding to hormone receptors. These chemicals cause damage to tissue that disrupts insulin sensitivity and glucose balance, accelerates aging, causes infertility, creates brain dysfunction and disturbs leptin, the weight and appetite regulating hormone. Besides disrupting body balance, these substances cause our bodies to store fat. Our bodies store toxins in the fat cells. Research shows that obesogens can even alter your genes.

We are exposed every day to xenoestrogens, which have been linked to prostate and breast cancer, infertility and widespread thyroid disorders.

You will want to avoid and limit your exposure to xenoestrogens as much as possible to prevent estrogen dominance and extra body fat, and to reduce any possible risk of estrogen dominant cancers. Researchers warn that endocrine disruptors such as xenoestrogens can trigger hormonal changes in the body that may not show up for decades.

## Hidden sources of estrogen disruptors (xenoestrogens)

* Artificial air fresheners, styrofoam products
* Food additives and preservatives, oxidized vegetable oils
* Household cleaners, detergents, car exhaust
* Conventional, non-organic foods
* Oral contraceptives and prescription drugs
* Paints, lacquers and solvents
* Parabens and triclosan
* Personal care products
* Pesticides, herbicides, fertilizers: Hormone disruptors in these chemicals have been linked to breast cancer, infertility, low sperm counts, genital deformities and early menstruation, as well as diabetes and obesity.
* Phthalates: found in food packaging, lotion, hair spray, nail polish, shampoo
* Plant estrogens (processed soy)
* Plastics: bisphenol-A (BPA) and bisphenol-S (BPS), found in canned goods, water bottles, food wrap and dental sealants
* Thermal receipts that come out of gas pumps, ATM machines and cash registers

See *Chapter 7* for more on obesogens.

## Label awareness

Protect yourself from chemicals that mimic estrogen. Get in the habit of reading the list of ingredients on all personal care products, cosmetics and cleaning products.

It's important to recognize that whatever you spread on your skin can be absorbed into your blood stream and potentially cause serious damage over time. Many antiperspirants and lotions we slather on our skin contain parabens. Parabens are an obesogen, and a direct cause of estrogen overload that will inhibit fat loss (see *Chapter 7*).

Opt for natural products that you trust.

## *Revolution Solutions* to reduce estrogen overload

* Avoid canned foods and water in plastic bottles.
* Replace conventional animal protein with organic, grass-fed and free-range animal protein as much as possible.
* Eat plenty of leafy greens such as kale, arugula and watercress, and cruciferous vegetables such as broccoli, brussel sprouts, cauliflower and cabbage. These foods contain compounds that promote a healthy estrogen metabolism.
* Eliminate consumption of vegetable oils and processed soy products.
* Enjoy some walnuts. Phytosterols, found in walnuts, bind to and block estrogen receptors.
* Estrogen-blockers can be beneficial for lowering estrogen and helpful for cellulite. These include green tea extract (EGCG), DIM, calcium D glucarate and sulphoraphane.
* Increase soluble fiber intake. Fiber excretes xenoestrogens from the body *and* decreases insulin secretion.
* Keep insulin levels low. Increase insulin sensitivity (see page 20).
* Opt for natural personal care products and cleaning goods.
* Wash your hands after handing ATM, gasoline or cash register receipts, or refuse to accept them.
* Store foods in glass or ceramic containers.
* Use natural pest control in your home and garden, such as soapy water, cayenne pepper, boric acid or oil of eucalyptus.

You can safely metabolize and excrete excess estrogen through a healthy diet, optimizing your liver's detoxification abilities and the quantity and quality of healthy flora in your gut.

# Ghrelin

Ghrelin is a hormone produced mainly by the stomach and pancreas that stimulates hunger. It is an important hormone in regulating body weight. Ghrelin levels increase before meals, stimulating appetite, and lower after eating a meal.

Ghrelin levels are positively related to stress hormones. Individuals suffering from lack of sleep or anorexia, and those who skip meals, particularly breakfast, usually have higher levels of ghrelin. Ghrelin levels usually rise when a person restricts calories too much, which leads to regaining the weight that was lost through calorie restriction. When ghrelin levels remain elevated, your brain is activated to eat more sweet and fatty foods.

Ghrelin can be stabilized by getting a minimum of six to eight hours of restful sleep, practicing stress management techniques and exercising. You can keep this appetite-stimulating hormone from raging out of control by eating a breakfast that is higher in protein. This will lower post-meal levels of ghrelin far greater than a breakfast high in carbohydrates. Consuming a high-fiber diet of fruits and vegetables also helps reduce ghrelin after a meal.

# Leptin

Leptin is a hormone released by fat cells that plays an important role in appetite control, metabolism and fat loss. In Greek, the translation of leptin means "thin." Leptin sends signals to your cells that reduce hunger, increase fat burning and minimize fat storage. Levels rise, communicating to your brain that you're full – that is, if your cells are communicating properly and can hear this message. There is a favorable fat burning environment when leptin levels are within normal healthy ranges. Over time, if your leptin levels are consistently elevated, your body will develop leptin resistance, similar to insulin resistance. Eating a diet high in grains, carbohydrates, fructose and sugar leads to leptin resistance.

The sugars metabolize into fat, which is then stored in your fat cells. This triggers a surge in leptin causing you to become leptin resistant, which nullifies the signal to stop eating and burning fat. The end result: you remain hungry. You crave more sugar and your body stores more fat than ever.

According to research from Monash University in Australia, leptin can substantially increase thermogenesis, helping to burn fat. When leptin levels rise, your appetite diminishes. Reduced levels of leptin have been shown to stimulate appetite. Crash diets and very low calorie diets lower your leptin levels to an unhealthy level and damage your metabolism, creating an environment to store body fat. In addition, thyroid hormones are disrupted, and the fat storing stress hormone, cortisol, rises.

A study in the *International Journal of Obesity Related Metabolism Disorders* found that just three days of eating a carb-heavy diet led to a 28 percent increase in leptin levels, whereas a diet consisting primarily of calories from fat had no effect on leptin.

Leptin can only boost one's metabolism so much. Leptin stimulates fatty acid oxidation and raises metabolism, but it does not completely offset chronic and excessive caloric intake from overeating and humungous portions. This causes fat cells to grow in size and number. When this happens, fat cells secrete more leptin that won't be used, causing leptin resistance.

The typical modern lifestyle contributes to leptin resistance: fast food; a diet high in grains, sugar and fructose; little or no exercise; excessive stress; and not getting enough restful sleep. Leptin resistance creates a problem for permanent fat loss, increasing both inflammation and visceral fat. Visceral fat is intra-abdominal hard fat that is located deep within the abdominal cavity where it pads the spaces between organs like your liver and heart. Subcutaneous fat, on the other hand, is found just beneath the skin – the fat you can pinch. Subcutaneous fat deposits correlate with circulating levels of leptin.

*Revolution Solutions* **to prevent leptin resistance**

* Reduce subcutaneous and visceral belly fat
* Avoid severe calorie restriction
* Eliminate lectins, specifically those from cereals and grains
* Limit fructose which inhibits leptin receptors
* Get seven to nine hours of sleep every night
* Follow the *Fat Loss Revolution* eating plan

## Adiponectin

Adiponectin is a protein hormone produced in the fat cells that helps break down fats (fatty acids) and regulate sugar (glucose) levels.

Adiponectin is also an anti-inflammatory, insulin-sensitizing marker. Its known benefits are mainly reducing the risk of diabetes and helping to redistribute fat away from unhealthy areas, such as the liver and belly.

Levels of this hormone are inversely related to how much body fat a person has, and are affected by the foods you eat and pharmaceutical drugs you take, including statin drugs.

Adiponectin improves insulin sensitivity and glucose uptake, communicating to your body to burn fat as fuel.

Higher levels of adiponection increase thermogenesis. Obesity is related to lower levels of adiponectin. In combination with leptin, adiponectin has been shown to completely reverse insulin resistance.

In a study of healthy adults, consumption of a Mediterranean diet was associated with increased levels of adiponectin.

Adiponectin levels can be boosted naturally with omega-3 fatty acids, magnesium and a low carbohydrate diet that includes more nuts, seeds, fresh vegetables and leafy greens.

## Hormones – Key Points to Remember

* Hormones do not act independently. Hormones work in synergy.

* Fat weight gain is caused by hormone imbalances. Balancing your hormones is a major factor to lasting fat loss.

* Exercising and dieting for fat loss will not make a difference unless insulin and cortisol are balanced.

* Insulin is the number one hormone to control for fat loss.

* You control your insulin levels by what you choose to eat.

* Determine your hormone levels with lab testing.

* Hormone response is influenced by the sleep you get, the stress you experience, your exercise program and the foods you eat.

* Diet, lifestyle, intelligent exercise and supplementation (the "four powers" from *The Power of 4*) all assist in balancing hormones.

* Balancing hormones takes time. It is not a quick-fix and does not happen overnight.

# CHAPTER 3

## A HEALTHY METABOLISM FOR A HOT 'N HEALTHY BODY

Y ou're doing everything right – you're exercising and eating a healthy diet, yet your results have come to a dead stop. You've reached a dreaded plateau. How frustrating! The problem may be a damaged metabolism.

### Do you have a damaged metabolism?

The definition of metabolism according to Diana Schwarzbein, M.D., founder of The Schwarzbein Principle Institute, is the combined effects of all the chemical reactions that continuously occur within your body on a daily basis.

Metabolism is how efficiently and effectively your body burns calories. It involves all the processes by which your body breaks down and uses food, water and air to function and maintain life. The rate of metabolism is very specific to each individual. Some people have a supercharged, high-octane, fast metabolism, and others have a snail-pace metabolism.

Metabolic efficiency depends on your mitochondria, which are the tiny powerhouse, energy factories in all of your cells. Dr. Mark Hyman, M.D., author of *Ultrametabolism,* defines metabolic rate as the "rate at which mitochondria transform food and oxygen into energy." That rate is influenced by your age, body composition, genetics and hormone function.

When you have a damaged metabolism, you will have a difficult time achieving an ideal body composition even though you're exercising and eating a clean diet. This is known as weight loss resistance. Any metabolic imbalance in the body can instigate weight loss resistance. A damaged metabolism does not happen overnight; therefore, healing a damaged metabolism takes time.

## Factors that cause a damaged metabolism

* Depression

* Digestive dysfunction

* Candida, parasites, H. pylori, infections

* Excessive consumption of grains, fructose, sugar, alcohol

* Food sensitivities

* Hormone imbalances: adrenal dysfunction, sluggish thyroid, insulin resistance

* Insufficient protein intake

* Overdoing cardiovascular exercise

* Prescription drugs and medications (antidepressants, beta blockers, glucocoticoid steroids)

* Skipping meals, fasting for extended periods, low-calorie diets, low fat diets and yo-yo dieting

* Sleep deprivation

* Toxic overload from chemical, obesogen and pesticide exposure

* Traumatic or prolonged psychological stress

All of these factors influence metabolism either directly or indirectly because metabolism is thought to be affected by lifestyle – the collaboration of many bodily functions and hormone balance – not just heredity, age and caloric intake. The *Fat Loss Revolution* will provide you with all of the information you need to heal and boost your metabolism naturally.

# Is a Calorie Just a Calorie?

The more calories you take in the fatter you get, and if you reduce your caloric intake the fat melts off. True or false? If that were 100 percent true, 500 calories of broccoli or 500 calories of chicken breast would be the same as 500 calories of doughnuts or jelly beans. Basically, you could consume a diet of just sugar without any adverse side effects. In reality, sugar is void of any nutritional value whatsoever, and creates an aggressive insulin response in the body. As a result, you would store more body fat, feel sick and eventually become unhealthy to the point of disease if continued long-term.

First, it may help to define a calorie. A calorie is a measurement of energy or heat obtained from a food source.

Many health-conscious people are obsessed with counting calories. The "calorie is a calorie" is commonly used by the processed food industry to explain that weight loss isn't really about what you eat, but about how many calories you eat. This can be very misleading.

While it is accurate that the balance of calories can influence whether you lose body fat or not, where the calories come from must be factored in. Food provides powerful information that influences hormones and whether you burn or store fat. Food choice determines your caloric balance based on your metabolic rate, satiety and the thermic effect of food (TEF). TEF is the energy expended by your body to consume and digest food.

Your body is fueled from three macronutrient sources: protein, carbohydrates and fat, and each have different thermic effects. The thermic effects for these nutrients are approximately 20-30 percent for protein, 5-10 percent for carbs and 2-3 percent for fat.

*Counting calories will not help you lose body fat if you're consuming the wrong type of calories.*

When comparing a diet high in carbohydrates to a diet that includes a higher amount of protein at the same amount of calories, the higher protein diet will produce a greater amount of fat loss due to the increased thermic effect of protein.

For every 100 protein calories you consume, your body needs 20 to 30 calories for digestion. On the other end of the spectrum, for every 100 calories of carbohydrate, your body expends only five to ten calories in digestion.

In addition, each macronutrient creates a different enzymatic and hormonal response in the body. Your thyroid, cortisol, insulin and other hormones are affected differently when you eat a bagel versus a piece of steak.

Whole foods and processed foods are not created equal. Just by consuming the nutrient-rich whole foods that nature intended for us to eat, you will rev up your metabolic rate and burn 50 percent more calories every day!

A 2011 study published in the *Journal of Clinical Nutrition* found that yo-yo dieting is associated with body weight excess and abdominal fat accumulation. In essence, when you restrict calories, your body thinks it's starving. This causes you to hang onto body fat and lose muscle. This behavior will cause a metabolic decline. This is why people who go on a low calorie diet regain all of the weight they lose plus some extra when they go off of the diet.

Another study in the *New England Journal of Medicine* revealed that hormones were disrupted and negatively affected in people on a 550 calorie diet, causing a surge in appetite and increased fat storage. In addition, metabolism is damaged due to the decline in resting metabolic rate (RMR) as a result of reduced caloric intake. Subjects experienced elevated levels of the hormone ghrelin, which as you recall in *Chapter 2,* is the hormone that stimulates hunger.

Different diets (e.g., a high-protein/low-carbohydrate diet versus a low-protein/high-carbohydrate diet) lead to different biochemical pathways that are not the same despite the fact that the high-protein/low-carb dieters consume considerably more calories.

If you recall in *Chapter 2* regarding hormones and their affect on fat loss, the quality and quantity of carbohydrates you consume has a direct influence on hormones ghrelin, the hunger hormone, and insulin, the fat-storing hormone.

In essence, the more processed, packaged and refined carbohydrates you eat, the more fat you store due to the surges in insulin and blood sugar fluctuations.

In his book *Good Calories, Bad Calories*, author Gary Taubes states, "If you had asked your mother or grandmother for diet tips, you might have heard, *'Every woman knows that carbohydrates are fattening.'*" In fact, that's from a 1963 article in the *British Journal of Nutrition*, co-authored by one of the leading nutritionists of the era. And, for the previous 100 years or so, conventional wisdom was that carbohydrate-rich foods such as bread, potatoes, pasta, rice, sweets and beer make us fat, and, by implication, foods rich in fat and protein do not.

1. *The calorie content of food is not a logical predictor for fat loss.*

2. *A protein calorie is NOT the same as a carbohydrate calorie.*

3. *Reducing carbohydrate consumption is a predictor for fat loss.*

4. *Although calories do matter, the hormonal impact of calories matters more.*

## Revolution Solutions and calories

It's important to shift your mindset from counting calories, and instead focus on eating a balanced, nutrient-dense, wholesome diet that includes quality protein and fiber from non-starchy vegetables and leafy greens at every meal.

Diets high in both protein and fiber will decrease the hormone ghrelin, reduce hunger and lower body fat levels compared to a diet high in carbohydrates or lower in fiber.

Inflammation, hormone levels, gut flora, satiety, energy and fat loss are all impacted by specific foods eaten. Fat loss is much easier when you choose to eat the right type of foods (see *Chapter14)* and include an intelligent exercise program (see *Chapter 11).*

This strategy is more favorable to creating a positive hormonal response and will increase your energy, stabilize your blood sugar, prevent fat accumulation and encourage fat loss. Plus, you will experience satiety, and sugar cravings will magically disappear.

When you choose to eat healthier foods and exercise intelligently, as suggested in the *Fat Loss Revolution,* losing body fat becomes natural and easy.

> *It is the hormonal response from certain calories that makes a difference for fat loss.*

# Jumpstart Your Metabolism – Eat Breakfast

Are you tempted to skip breakfast because you're not hungry in the morning? Are you rushing and hurrying about in the morning and just don't have time for breakfast? Are you like many Americans grabbing a bagel and coffee as you run out the door? If so, you're one step closer to downgrading your metabolism.

Skipping breakfast is a guaranteed recipe for gaining body fat and building insulin resistance, which can lead to type 2 diabetes. And, if you're recovering from adrenal fatigue, breakfast is especially important. What you choose to eat for breakfast is just as important. The first meal of your day will reflect how you think and feel the rest of the day. Harvard researchers have found that eating in the morning causes your brain to produce serotonin, which is a natural mood enhancer.

Katherine Tucker, Ph.D., professor of nutrition at Tufts University, says, "When you skip breakfast, you miss out on vital nutrients that promote peak cognition." A study published in the *American Journal of Clinical Nutrition* found that when women missed breakfast, they consumed more food the remainder of the day, and their cholesterol and insulin levels were negatively affected with a decrease in HDL, an increase in LDL and elevated insulin levels.

Another study from the University of Massachusetts Medical School conveyed that "people who skipped breakfast regularly were 450 percent more likely to be obese than individuals who ate breakfast."

Plain and simple: when you skip breakfast your hormones and your blood glucose are affected negatively, causing you to store more body fat. When blood glucose levels are low (hypoglycemia), or when the body has an impaired use of glucose, willpower will be impaired. Numerous studies confirm that low blood glucose levels and poor glucose use are associated with lack of self-control and emotional and behavioral problems.

A study in the *Journal of the Academy of Nutrition and Dietetics* found that women who do not skip meals lose up to eight pounds more versus women who skip meals.

Now that you're aware that skipping breakfast is not in your best interest, let's focus on selecting healthier choices for breakfast. What you choose to eat can be just as detrimental as not eating anything at all.

Consuming a bagel with a sugar-sweetened coffee drink, or sugar in a box of cereal with a banana and low-fat or non-fat milk are some of the worst choices for your morning meal, creating a metabolic nightmare. Although cereal or the coffee/bagel option may be convenient, the high-glycemic load of a bagel, cereal, low-fat or non-fat milk, a banana and juice causes a blood sugar roller coaster and activates an aggressive insulin response – the perfect blend if you want to get fatter, crash in the afternoon or end up with impaired blood sugar management long-term.

Most boxed cereals contain processed grains that are void of any nutrients and are full of sugar, chemical-laden dyes, soy, genetically engineered ingredients and a sprinkle of synthetic vitamins. And, the pasteurized milk poured on cereal is mostly sugar-water since the nutrients are killed off during the pasteurization process. Ultimately, what you end up with is a nutritionally-void, insulin-spiking meal, where your blood sugar increases rapidly followed by a sharp drop in your energy a couple of hours later. No wonder you crave a sugary caffeine jolt in the afternoon.

> *Nearly all grains act like sugar in the body, triggering inflammation, blood sugar imbalances and added body fat.*

## Let's talk coffee

You can enjoy your morning cup of coffee, as long as it's not the first thing in your body and not the only thing you consume for breakfast. Eat a nutrient-rich breakfast, and then brew a cup of joe. Just make sure to avoid the calorie-laden coffee beverages that are loaded with sugary syrups and artificial sweeteners. If you choose to drink coffee in the morning, opt for an organic whole bean brand of coffee and grind it yourself. Conventional coffee is highly sprayed with pesticides that can act as hormone disruptors.

## Breakfast solutions

Fuel your brain and body with a nourishing, well-balanced breakfast that includes a quality, organic protein source and soluble fiber from dark leafy greens, non-starchy vegetables or berries.

Protein, healthy fats and fiber will prevent blood sugar fluctuations, increase energy and metabolism, fuel your brain and eliminate cravings later in the day. In fact, the first 40 grams of protein you eat every day go to rebuild your immune system. If you are not rebuilding your immune system, you will have a hard time rebuilding your brain chemistry to be happy and think straight.

Protein initiates thermogenesis – energy production through heat/fat burning – and encourages increases in muscle mass. Protein is also rich in amino acids, the buildings blocks that help balance brain chemistry by boosting the levels of mood-regulating neurotransmitters (chemical messengers in the brain), specifically dopamine and acetylcholine. These neurotransmitters are beneficial for concentration, energy production and mood stabilization. See *Chapter 13* for more on the importance of protein.

Eating a nutrient-rich breakfast that includes a quality protein source and fiber will also reduce binge cravings later in the day and optimize cognitive function, elevate your mood and prevent that afternoon energy crash.

Adding some raw, organic nuts or seeds to your breakfast is another way to introduce healthy fats to your breakfast meal, provided you are not allergic to certain nuts or seeds. A study in *Nutrition and Metabolism* revealed that eating nuts at breakfast helps stabilize blood sugar and induce feelings of satiety versus the blood sugar roller coaster and hunger associated with a high-glycemic juice and toast breakfast.

Following are some delicious, protein-packed breakfast options that are sure to increase your energy, enhance cognition, boost your metabolism, decrease body fat and please your pallet.

Remember, there is no rule that says you must eat the typical American breakfast foods for breakfast.

**Protein–packed breakfast options.** Before breakfast, enjoy a cup of water with the fresh juice from a lemon or lime.

1.  Buffalo burger with salsa, handful of pine nuts, blackberries

2.  Eggs, chicken jalapeño sausage, sautéed spinach, avocado

3.  Mean 'n Green Protein Smoothie: kale, watercress, parsley, cucumber, green apple, ginger and fresh lime juice blended in a Vitamix or high-powered blender. Add ice, frozen berries, one tablespoon coconut oil, and a scoop of Protein Plus, Vital Whey or Whey Cool to create a balanced meal.

4.  Protein Smoothie: Chocolate coconut milk, chocolate Vital Whey protein powder, frozen raspberries, chia seeds and ice, blended. Enjoy with a handful of your favorite nuts or seeds.

5.  Organic quinoa flakes with coconut oil, cinnamon, pecans, and blueberries

6.  Chicken Apple Walnut Goodness: Sauté a chopped apple, chicken apple sausage and walnuts in coconut oil; sprinkle with cinnamon. (Courtesy of Evelyn Lambrecht)

*See Chapter 13 for more breakfast ideas.*

## Revolution Solutions to Heal a Damaged Metabolism

* Consume a balanced, whole-food diet found in the *Fat Loss Revolution*. Doing so will rev up your metabolic rate, and you will burn 50 percent more calories per day. In addition, you'll stabilize blood sugar, improve insulin sensitivity, prevent insulin resistance, preserve lean muscle tissue and lose more body fat faster.
* Balance hormones and correct nutritional deficiencies with lifestyle modifications and supplemental support to help rebuild the body.
* Eat a protein-packed breakfast every day. A fat loss tip from coach Charles Poliquin is for females to consume 40-50 grams of protein before lunch, and males to consume 60-70 grams of protein before lunch.
* Include a source of protein at breakfast, lunch and dinner to increase thermogenesis.
* Get 7-9 hours of quality sleep every night. The majority of growth hormone, a key anabolic hormone, is released during sleep and is critical for repairing the body.
* Build muscle with an intelligent strength training program (see *Chapter 11*).
* Manage stress and explore issues such as self-image, emotional connections with food and state-of-mind when eating.

When you make the appropriate nutrition and lifestyle changes as presented in the *Fat Loss Revolution*, your hormones will balance responsively and you will heal your metabolism. No question about it: repairing a damaged metabolism takes time, but with patience, perseverance and persistence, you will restore your metabolism and that troublesome fat will disappear. Stay focused on achieving optimal health instead of counting calories and the number on the scale, and the fat will melt away without obsessing about it.

> *Consistency is of utmost importance when healing a damaged metabolism.*

# CHAPTER 4

## ELIMINATING INFLAMMATION FOR A
## HOT 'N HEALTHY BODY

Inflammation is a silent killer. The cause of every degenerative disease of aging has been linked to chronic inflammation, including diabetes, arthritis, obesity, heart disease, cancer, Alzheimer's disease and Parkinson's disease.

### Put out the fire – inflammation and fat loss

Some level of inflammation is required in your body to stay healthy so tissue and wounds heal from infections, injuries, surgery or trauma. However, it is when the inflammatory response gets out of hand that inflammation causes problems.

### Common causes of inflammation

* Acute and chronic injuries
* Carbohydrate-heavy meals
* Chronic infections
* Consuming intolerant foods (see *Chapter 5*)
* Dehydration
* Diets with a high ratio of omega-6 to omega-3 essential fatty acids and with hydrogenated and trans-fats
* Digestive dysfunction and poor gut health
* Environmental: personal care products, petrochemicals, pesticides, air pollution, and toxic heavy metals
* Excessive or lack of exercise
* Heavy metal body burdens
* High-stress lifestyles
* Long-term use of birth control pills, NSAIDs or other drugs
* Sleep deprivation

Symptoms linked to an inflamed body may present as headaches, puffiness, bleeding gums, arthritis or a number of other health conditions.

An inflamed gut results in altered neurotransmitter production and excess cortisol. Long-term inflammation leads to destruction and damage of your cells, which accelerates the aging process. In fact, your body can be so inflamed yet you may not have any idea because you can't actually see it.

Inflammation may also be the reason you're hanging onto stubborn body fat. In fact, excess weight can itself be the cause of inflammation. When your body is inflamed, your efforts to lose body fat are futile and will come to a screeching halt no matter what you do.

You can control and prevent underlying causes of inflammation by changing your diet, healing your gut, managing stress and reducing exposure to environmental chemicals.

These approaches take time, discipline, consistency and energy, but they are extremely effective at reducing, minimizing and eliminating inflammation. My intention and focus is to prevent the initiation and sources of excess inflammation from happening in the first place, and then guide you toward controlling and reducing inflammation.

### Revolution Solution – start with a dietary shift

The solution to controlling and eliminating inflammation starts with diet, nutrition and eliminating inflammatory foods. Certain foods, nutrients and herbs have powerful anti-inflammatory effects.

The initial approach to reduce inflammation is to start by healing and restoring gut dysfunction. Two-thirds of the body's defenses are in the gastrointestinal (GI) tract, yet it is often the last place traditional practitioners look to determine the root cause of any dysfunction or disease (see *Chapter 6*)

The process of healing the gut starts with the elimination of intolerant and pro-inflammatory foods, specifically sugar, polyunsaturated vegetable oils, processed dairy, gluten, wheat and non-wheat grains and genetically-modified foods (see *Chapter 7*).

According to Mark Hyman, M.D., "the two most common dietary sources of inflammation in the 21st century are sugar (and refined carbohydrates) and hidden food allergens (perhaps most important, gluten)."

A dietary shift must be initiated to avoid other inflammatory foods including corn, soy, sugar, trans-fats, omega-6 fats (vegetable oils), nightshade vegetables (potato, tomato, eggplant), and sugary beverages. Regular consumption of these inflammatory foods increases your risk for insulin resistance, leptin resistance and other conditions, making it impossible to lose body fat.

Other items to be aware of that create excess inflammation include food additives such as MSG, sulfites, aspartame and other artificial sweeteners, high-fructose corn syrup, trans-fats, GMOs, artificial colorings and preservatives – all of which play a major role in the inflammatory process of every cell in your body (see *Chapter 7*).

Going back to what was discussed about insulin, keep in mind that anything that creates a high insulin response, such as processed carbohydrates and sugar, promotes inflammation.

Overall, eating foods that your body is sensitive to or intolerant of creates inflammation in the intestinal tract by stimulating the immune system to attack your cells instead of healing them.

The key to identifying inflammation is to listen to your own body and pay attention to your individual symptoms and the foods that tend to fuel an inflammatory response within your own body. This is where the importance of keeping a food journal can be beneficial.

## Revolution Solutions to put out the fire

**Consume an anti-inflammatory diet.** For the majority of individuals, a low-protein and carbohydrate-heavy diet is one that is inflammatory.

Include plenty of dark leafy greens, non-starchy vegetables and berries, which are very low in sugar and a rich source of flavonoids, carotenoids and antioxidants, nutrients that contain anti-inflammatory properties. Opt for a wide range of colorful fruits and vegetables that are fresh or frozen. Buy organic as often as possible.

Raspberries, blueberries, strawberries, peaches, nectarines, oranges, pink grapefruit, red grapes, plums, pomegranates, cranberries, blackberries, cherries, apples and pears are all excellent low sugar choices as opposed to the higher sugar found in most tropical fruits.

Vegetables and dark, leafy greens contain vitamins, minerals, bioflavonoids, polyphenols and antioxidants that are all necessary to decrease inflammation and limit free-radical production in the body. Free radical production, like inflammation, caters to cell destruction rather than healthy cell formation.

Include organic, hormone-free, antibiotic-free, wild seafood, oily fish, meat and poultry. Wild salmon is especially anti-inflammatory. When you consume commercially-raised protein sources in which the animals are fed a diet of grain, corn, processed soy, hormones and antibiotics, your digestive system suffers. Commercially-raised protein sources promote inflammation and cause hormone disruption.

Fats are an excellent anti-inflammatory source provided they are healthy fats. You'll want to add ample amounts of healthy fats from wild fish, avocado, raw nuts, chia seeds, flax and other seeds, pastured butter, coconut oil and olive oil to your anti-inflammatory *Fat Loss Revolution* eating plan.

Onions, garlic, parsley, rosemary, cinnamon, turmeric and ginger; red wine; green and white teas and cocoa are also other powerful natural anti-inflammatory agents. Be sure to include these options into your new plan as well.

Cultured or fermented foods boost the immune system and fight inflammation. Aloe vera, which is an amazing food plant with potent anti-inflammatory properties, is also highly beneficial for healing an inflamed gut and a natural cure for constipation.

**Rule out hidden food intolerances** and adverse reactions to specific foods that drive inflammation. Keep a daily food journal.

Refer to *Chapter 5* for the top offending and intolerant foods and how they inhibit fat loss.

> *To reduce inflammation and encourage greater fat loss, remember these two key points:*
>
> 1. *Avoid high-density carbohydrates, vegetable oils, and all processed, packaged and fast foods.*
>
> 2. *Eliminate intolerant foods from your diet.*

**Stay hydrated** and drink quality, filtered water to help put out the inflammatory fire. White, green and oolong teas are rich in catechins, antioxidant compounds that reduce inflammation. Just make sure the tea is organic to avoid high pesticides.

**Balanced blood sugar** and stable insulin levels are crucial for reducing inflammation. Processed sugars and other high-glycemic starches increase inflammation, just as they raise blood sugar. An individual with blood sugar issues almost always has some sort of inflammatory gut dysfunction.

**Sleep.** A number of studies have reported associations between disrupted sleep, sleep deprivation and increased inflammation. Alterations in sleep due to lifestyle factors, the aging process and diseased states have all been associated with increases in a range of inflammatory markers. Refer to *Chapter 5* for *Revolution Solutions* for Insomnia.

The physical body repairs between the hours of 10:00 p.m. and 2:00 a.m., and emotional and spiritual regeneration occurs between the hours of 2:00 a.m. and 6:00 a.m. Seven to nine hours of quality, restful sleep during these hours can undo the effects of inflammatory response.

**Rule out heavy metal body burdens.** Heavy metals are toxic to the body and trigger an inflammatory response. Inflammation is a symptom of heavy metal toxicity which often goes undetected. Inflammation becomes chronic when the body has to continuously fight off repeated offenders, such as Candida, H.pylori, or heavy metal toxicity.

**Chronic infections,** including HSV, CMB, EBV, pneumonia, flu, Chlamydia, pneumonia, mycoplasma, periodontal and H. Pylori all promote excess inflammation and should be ruled out.

**Gut pathogens.** Often overlooked when it comes to fat loss and many other health conditions are intestinal pathogens such as parasites and/or Candida, which lead to systemic inflammation.

Adhere to the dietary suggestions found in the *Fat Loss Revolution* plus garlic, oregano and cultured foods will starve the bugs, yeast and fungus. Encourage healing with a supplemental protocol to kill the pathogens with specific nutritional supplements and rebuild the intestinal environment with pre– and probiotics. *Saccharomyces boulardii* is a probiotic that supports the environment of the GI tract, protects against intestinal dysbiosis, is effective against Candida overgrowth and prevents Candida from forming.

**Sedentary lifestyles** promote inflammation. Start moving your body daily by doing the *Fat Loss Revolution* workouts (see *Chapter 11*).

**Physical, mental and emotional stress** is another contribution to the inflammatory cascade. Managing stress and learning how to cope with emotional pain can help restore balance within the body.

**Environmental causes of inflammation** you're exposed to everyday can trigger an excess of inflammation. Many individuals fail to recognize that personal care products, pesticides, air pollution and toxic heavy metals all create an inflammatory burden on the body.

**Nutrient "flame fighters."** Antioxidants and other supplements are beneficial in lowering inflammation and decreasing oxidative stress. My favorite inflammation flame fighters, listed in order of priority, include:
* Vitamin D: Both obesity and inflammation decrease the conversion of sunlight to vitamin D.
* Curcumin, a nutrient found in turmeric
* Omega-3 fatty acids
* Magnesium
* Proteolytic enzymes
* Coenzyme Q10
* Quercetin
* Olive oil
* Probiotics
* Ginger
* Cocoa and cacao
* Green tea extract (EGCG)
* Hydrochloric acid (HCL)
* Resveratrol
* Aged garlic

**Balance hormones.** Fluctuating hormone levels such as insulin, cortisol, testosterone, estrogen and progesterone play a role in age-related inflammation. Symptoms of chronic inflammation tend to become more evident during and after menopause as women become more sensitive to inflammation after menopause.

**Test fasting insulin and C-reactive protein (CRP).** CRP level is used as a marker of inflammation in the arteries. Fasting insulin is a test that screens for diabetes and heart disease, but it's also a marker for inflammation.

# CHAPTER 5

## LET'S GET HONEST ABOUT FLAT ABS FOR A
## HOT 'N HEALTHY BODY

L iposuction, endless abdominal crunches and exercises that target the abs, the latest infomercial gadget...all promise flatter, well-defined mid-sections. In reality, these common misconceptions deliver very little to no return on your investment.

Belly fat is composed of two different types of fat, subcutaneous or visceral. Visceral fat is hard, intra-abdominal fat located deep within the abdominal wall where it pads the spaces between organs such as your liver and heart. Subcutaneous fat, on the other hand, is found just beneath the skin, the fat you can grab or pinch with calipers.

In order to see definition in your abs, you must lower your overall body fat percentage. Seventy-five to 80 percent of your ability to reduce excess body fat and visually see defined abs is influenced by the foods you choose to eat. The remaining 20-25 percent is related to addressing any reactions you may have to specific foods; an intelligently designed exercise program; optimal hormone balance with specific attention to cortisol and insulin; genetics; and other lifestyle factors including stress and sleep.

Certain foods have been found to specifically target abdominal fat. According to a study at Wake Forest Baptist Medical Center, soluble fiber found in fruits and especially vegetables directly affects midsection fat. Participants in the study reduced visceral fat 3.7 percent simply by consuming an additional 10 grams of soluble fiber per day.

A diet that includes a sufficient amount of quality, organic protein not only encourages greater fat loss, but will also decrease intra-abdominal adipose tissue (belly fat) and stabilize blood sugar.

Including healthy monounsaturated fats in your diet such as avocado, nuts, seeds and extra-virgin olive oil are also effective in diminishing abdominal fat. Other belly blasting items include coconut oil, green tea, water and raw, organic chocolate that contains at least 70 percent cacao.

The abdominal muscles are primarily fast twitch muscles, which means the exercise prescription that the abdominal muscles respond best to is one that focuses on overloading the muscle with lower reps and higher intensity. Lower repetitions and heavier weight loads will activate fast twitch muscle fibers. In a University of Virginia study, middle-aged women who exercised at higher intensity lost more abdominal fat than women who exercised at lower intensity.

## Menopause and belly fat

Women tend to struggle with unexplained belly fat as they approach menopause or during peri-menopause as they experience a change in the way fat accumulates in their mid-section. This unexplained belly fat is caused by genetics and hormonal changes.

A woman may struggle with fluctuating estrogen and progesterone levels during peri-menopause, or experience a decline in estrogen after menopause. What they have done in the past to manage their weight and body composition no longer seems to be effective. Menopause weight gain is just another indication that your system is out of balance, particularly cortisol and insulin imbalances. When estrogen production fluctuates or declines, this causes profound effects on memory and mood, ability to maintain a normal weight or lose weight, and overall sense of well-being.

As production of estradiol (estrogen made in the ovaries) declines or is insufficient, higher levels of insulin and cortisol occur, resulting in excess mid-section fat accumulation. Insulin increases fat production and cortisol stores fat in the midsection. The higher your insulin and cortisol levels are, the more belly fat you will have. The only way to remedy the excess belly fat is to balance insulin and cortisol.

Consuming a high-fat diet triggers the production of aldehyde dehydrogenase 1 (Aldh1a1), an enzyme that produces retonic acid, a hormone that stimulates the production of visceral fat, particularly in women.

Consumption of high-fat, heavy carbohydrate and sugary foods sets off a chemical reaction in women, causing them to store more fat in their abdomens, explaining why women often gain excess belly fat after menopause.

## The *Revolution Solution* for balancing hormones

Balancing your hormones, specifically insulin and cortisol, must be prioritized to reduce excess belly fat. It is also important to get sufficient sleep, detoxify periodically, have healthy functioning digestion and flora in the gut, and implement stress management techniques. Adopting the *Fat Loss Revolution* lifestyle and diet, along with the workout programs found in *Chapter 11,* when done consistently, will shrink your waistline, reduce belly fat and flatten your abs in just 12 weeks, resulting in a "Hot 'n Healthy Body"!

## Are Food Sensitivities and Food Intolerances Making You Fat?

Food really is a drug. You may be completely unaware that a specific food or food item you're consuming is responsible for creating inflammation in your body, elevating cortisol levels and preventing you from losing body fat. Look at the chart below. Do any of these symptoms or conditions resonate with you? If so, it is highly probable that the cause is related to the food(s) you're eating.

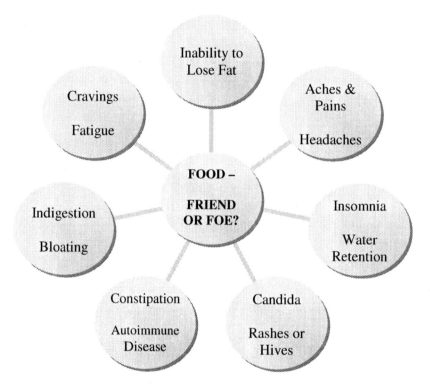

One of the leading causes of obesity and an inability to lose body fat is related to food sensitivity or a food intolerance, an adverse reaction to food(s) that occurs over time. Many individuals are completely unaware that eating wheat, dairy, soy or any other trigger food is the root cause of why they're not feeling well, and despite their ongoing efforts, they cannot lose weight.

**Food allergy** is an IgE reaction of the body's immune system to a food or food ingredient that it recognizes as "foreign." A true food allergy is driven by an IgE antibody and can cause tingling in the mouth; hives; swelling of the lips, face, tongue and throat; trouble breathing; and dizziness or fainting. It can also cause nausea, vomiting, cramping and diarrhea, signs and symptoms that happen with a food intolerance as well. Food allergy rates are higher for children, African-Americans, males and people with asthma.

**Food sensitivity** is a *non*-IgE reaction (IgG, IgA, IgM) in which an individual experiences an adverse reaction over time to a food, food ingredient or additive. A food sensitivity usually involves the digestive system and the immune system sensing a food as a foreign invader. You can probably eat small amounts of the food *without* an immediate reaction. However, if you continue eating foods your body considers harmful, inflammation increases and your immune system is compromised, as shown by the many symptoms listed on page 64.

**Food intolerance** is when your body is unable to break down, assimilate, digest or absorb a food, food ingredient or additive due to a lack of enzymes or insufficient hydrochloric acid production.

Food sensitivities and intolerances have increased 20 percent in the last ten years. Nearly 80 percent of the population is sensitive or intolerant to one or more foods. Eating the same foods over and over, day after day after day, is one of the most sure-fire methods that guarantee you will develop a food intolerance. Many women have been sensitive to certain foods for years, but only realize it during midlife after a decline in estrogen levels. Food sensitivities and intolerances are a primary cause of fatigue, emotional problems, bloating, inflammation and excess body fat.

Do you crave or are you addicted to any specific food(s)? If so, chances are quite high you are more than likely intolerant or sensitive to it. Eating intolerant foods is toxic to your system and increases inflammation in the body, which causes you to retain water and inhibit fat loss.

**Top trigger foods responsible for 90 percent of food reactions**

| | |
|---|---|
| Wheat and gluten | Milk, dairy and casein |
| Peanuts and tree nuts | Sugar / Artificial sweeteners |
| Soy | Fish and shellfish |
| Corn | Eggs, specifically egg white |

In addition, many people are intolerant to MSG; food dyes; beer, wine and cocktail mixes; and sulfites and other preservatives. As we get older, foods that never bothered us before, like dairy and wheat, may trigger chronic low-grade indigestion or other symptoms. Even healthy foods can cause problems and reactions.

*Revolution Solutions.* Completely eliminate all wheat, gluten, soy, cow's milk and pasteurized dairy products, corn and all artificial sweeteners. Supplements and protein powders that contain additives, high-fructose corn syrup, artificial sweeteners and fillers should also be removed from the diet.

Initially, when you eliminate these foods, you may experience temporary withdrawal symptoms similar to withdrawal from other addictive substances like caffeine, nicotine, drugs and alcohol. But the payoff is worth it.

You will experience deeper sleep; less bloating, brain fog, fatigue, aches and pains; relief from inflammation; increased mental clarity; a surge in energy; reduced stress and lower cortisol levels; clearer, healthier looking skin; and a flatter belly.

To avoid food sensitivities and intolerances, it's important to rotate the foods you eat every day and read the list of ingredients on every product. Even healthy foods when eaten day after day after day can cause a reaction.

On a rotation diet, a food is only eaten once every four days. As a result, if you have eggs on Monday, you will not eat eggs again until Friday.

Keep a daily food journal of everything you eat and drink. Doing so helps identify trigger foods and keeps you accountable of how often you are consuming them.

Consider a self-test. Eliminate the top trigger foods from your diet. If you do not develop any symptoms within a month of quitting the foods, then the responsible food is within the list. Start introducing one food at a time, and wait three days to see if you develop any type of reaction.

Start tracking your food intake and amount eaten on a piece of paper you carry in your purse or pocket, or in a spiral notebook, an app on your smart phone, a word document, or a computer program. Always carry your food log with you. Be honest and consistent, and record everything that goes into your mouth.

> *Those who journal what they eat tend to **lose twice as much weight** and make much healthier food choices compared to those who do not keep a journal.*
>
> *A food journal is a great tool that can help identify food(s) that your body is sensitive to or intolerant of.*

If you have persistent health issues that don't seem to get better no matter what you do, you may want to consider a thorough screening with the lab work listed on the next page, even if you get a negative result on your self-elimination test.

## Testing for food intolerances and sensitivities

Most labs performing food allergy tests identify the presence of IgE- and IgG-type antibodies. A non-IgE reaction test, such as IgG and IgA tests, is different than a food allergy (skin prick) test (IgE).

An IgE response is normally associated with the allergic response to food(s). Foods that stimulate elevated IgE responses are those that cause serious health problems and should be completely avoided.

IgG and IgA tests rule out intolerant food(s) and identify immune responses to specific food(s). Foods that stimulate IgG production are foods that should be eliminated temporarily in order to evaluate the individual's response.

It has been suggested that up to 90 percent of food allergies are IgG-mediated. For this reason, it is important to test for the presence of both of these antibody types.

Another test to consider is LEP/MRT. This blood test is an accurate and comprehensive test that can also help identify food sensitivities. CBC, HbA1C, Human leukocyte antigen (HLA), genetic testing and IgA stool titers are other tests to consider.

## The Skinny-mini on Stress & Sleep for a Hot 'n Healthy Body

What do stress and sleep have to do with fat loss? Plenty! An individual who is sleep-deprived and chronically stressed out is an individual who will age faster and have a difficult time losing body fat. Combine that with an unhealthy diet, imbalanced hormones and zero exercise, and you have the perfect recipe for obesity.

## Got stress?

Stress is almost always a reaction to an emotional situation. Stress is not the situation itself, but your mental and emotional reaction to your perception of the stressor. Your stress level directly influences how you feel at the beginning or the end of your day, your health, your relationships and your ability to lose body fat. While short bursts of stress are actually beneficial, it is the continual, long-term, chronic stress that is damaging to your health and your waistline.

Stress can be defined as either sudden, short-term (acute) or long-term (chronic).

**Acute stress** is the immediate reaction to threat, challenge or scare, commonly known as the "fight-or-flight response" (see *Chapter 2*). A single episode of acute stress can be any situation that is perceived, even subconsciously or falsely, as a danger. Acute stress usually does not cause problems for healthy people.

**Examples of acute stress:**

* Job interview
* Fender-bender
* Noise
* Crowds
* Hang gliding
* Sitting in traffic
* Dental appointment

While mild, acute stress can actually be beneficial, motivating and energizing you, the problem occurs when acute stressors continue over time.

**Chronic stress** is the grinding, prolonged stress that wears people down day after day, year after year. This persistent stress is harder to handle and can lead to health problems such as leaky gut syndrome, adrenal burnout, headaches, insomnia and stalling fat loss. Chronic stress destroys minds, bodies and lives.

**Examples of chronic stress:**
* Loneliness
* Persistent financial worries
* Hidden, unmanaged food sensitivities or infections
* Staying in an unhappy relationship, job or career that is not nourishing

## Stress and hormone dysfunction

Chronic stress causes a continuous production of stress hormones into your bloodstream and body leading to adrenal burnout. When high amounts of the stress hormone, cortisol, are released, production of sex hormones decline and instead produce more stress hormones. Studies have shown that this continuous release of stress hormones can actually kill nerve cells in animals and can probably do the same in humans.

In excess, cortisol is destructive to your brain and your body. When cortisol goes up, DHEA goes down and telomeres shorten. Telomeres are sections of genetic DNA-protein material at the end of each chromosome, and like the plastic caps on the end of shoelaces, they serve a protective function. When telomeres shorten, the cell's lifespan shortens and the chromosomes become damaged, resulting in DNA destruction, which causes biological or cellular aging.

Shortened telomeres have been linked to increased risk of cancers, heart disease, dementia and mortality. Women with the highest levels of perceived stress have the shortest telomeres, indicating that they have a cell age ten years ahead of their biological age (see *Chapter 2*).

Too much cortisol ultimately reduces muscle mass, weakens digestive function, elevates blood sugar, increases the likelihood of food reactions and causes excess fat accumulation around the hips and abdominal area.

According to the Study of Women's Health Across the Nation, the more stress in a woman's life, the greater her weight. Another study in *Molecular Psychiatry* found that women are more sensitive to the stress hormone, cortisol, and are less able to adapt when levels are high.

There are over 1,400 chemical reactions that occur in the body as a result of excess stress. Corticotrophin releasing factor (CRF), which acts as both a hormone and a neurotransmitter, is activated during stress and attaches to receptors on cell membranes in the brain's alarm center. This leads to an aroused mental state. Compared with females, male brains need more CRF to become agitated. Researchers discovered that in males, the receptors retreat inside the cells, eluding CRF to minimize stress. Even in the absence of any stress, the researchers found the female stress-signaling system more sensitive in the females. Perhaps this is one well-known reason why women have higher incidences of anxiety and depression.

Long-term, chronic stress suppresses, rather than stimulates, your immune system, increasing your risk for infectious disease. It can also impair memory and cognitive function, and increase anxiety and the risk of depression. It has been linked to cellular and accelerated brain aging. Chronic stress also increases body fat.

Stress is also linked to overconsumption of certain types of food, particularly processed carbohydrates, sugar and unhealthy fats.

A study conducted by researchers at the University of Liverpool gave participants unlimited access to chocolate after a stressful event. Females proved more likely to overconsume the chocolate in response to stress, eating up to 120 grams of chocolate in one sitting.

When all is said and done, an inability to tolerate stress leads to physical breakdown and emotional overeating, and inhibits fat loss.

Stress affects a number of bodily processes, including:

* A reduction in the amino acid, L-tryptophan, which in turn decreases serotonin levels. Serotonin is an important neurotransmitter that regulates mood, sleep and appetite, and affects learning and memory. Symptoms of low serotonin include anxiety, depression, sugar cravings and insomnia.
* How your metabolism stores fat, sending excess flab to your belly where it affects vital organs.
* A decline in secretory IgA, antibodies produced in the intestinal tract. This causes digestive dysfunction and creates a prime environment for pathogens like Candida, parasites and bacterial infections to breed.
* Immune dysfunction.
* A flood of sugar and fat into the blood stream, increasing risk of diabetes, heart disease and many other adverse health conditions.

**Sources of stress** and anxiety affect our bodies and lives:

* Physical stress – digestive distress, imbalanced hormones, food intolerances, chronic illness, excess body fat, toxic overload, processed and GE foods, chronic infections
* Mental stress – economy, jobs, finances, retirement
* Emotional stress – relationships, divorce, hormone imbalances, depression, anxiety, low self esteem, negative thoughts
* Environmental stress – environmental toxins, chemicals, electromagnetic stress from computers, cell phones, microwave ovens
* Spiritual stress – unhealthy beliefs
* Although stress is life and life is stress, the key is to build resiliency when challenges arise. Stress management is learning to identify and recognize the best way to respond to challenges that will inevitably occur in everyone's lives.

## Simple "Stress–less" solutions

**Breathe.** Become aware of your breathing patterns. Deep breathing is easy to do and can be done anytime and anywhere. And, it's free! The breath is the foundation of de-stressing and healing. It is revitalizing and energizing to every cell in your body. Deep, full breathing brings in more oxygen, which causes a release of endorphins that create feelings of happiness, peace and calm by shifting the autonomic nervous system from overstimulation to relaxation.

Allow yourself five minutes in the morning and five minutes in the evening to focus on deep belly breathing. When you breathe deeply using the diaphragm, you consume a full breath into the belly as opposed to using your lungs and rib cage. When you take in a deep, full breath, your belly inflates as you inhale and deflates as you exhale. It is very similar to that of a newborn infant's breath: their little bellies push out and in as they breathe.

Empty your mind of your day-to-day activities and focus on a one- to five-word phrase that resonates with you. Repeat it over and over again, or surrender into the silence. Imagine yourself breathing in harmony and relaxation, and as you exhale let go of all stress and negativity. Envision a peaceful environment such as the ocean or a beautiful garden full of colorful flowers. Studies show this lowers blood pressure, boosts immune function, releases healing hormones on a cellular level, increases creativity and productivity, and enhances your ability to handle stressful situations as they arise.

**Meditate.** A proven stress buster, meditation positively charges the brain. A simple form of meditation is to focus your attention on your breath while repeating a phrase, prayer or mantra to shift the autonomic nervous system. We have to practice discipline of the mind to get rid of the "monkey mind." Start with just two to five minutes of meditation in the morning and early evening.

**Get out in nature.** Studies show that our environment contributes up to 70 percent of our stress. Children and adults are spending more and more time indoors with artificial lighting. As a result, there are more health problems such as ADHD and obesity.

Environmental psychologists have demonstrated that contact with nature restores attention and mental focus and helps the mind to recover from mental fatigue. Spending time in nature creates a positive effect on mental and physical well-being and induces a sense of connectedness, spirituality, meaning and purpose. Research says that even gazing out the window at a garden or looking at a photo of a natural setting can reduce stress. Schedule more time at the beach, the mountains or a tree-filled park.

**Avoid sugar, white flour and processed, packaged foods.** These items exacerbate stress and increase oxidation. Eliminating processed, packaged foods will also help regulate insulin levels so your blood sugar level stays consistent instead of rapidly rising and falling in response to the sugary, processed foods. When blood sugar drops, adrenaline is released to compensate for the lack of energy, thereby increasing stress and anxiety. It is important not to keep trigger foods in your home to avoid giving into the temptation to reach for these when you're experiencing anxiety or stress.

**Drink water.** Many people are chronically dehydrated, which places tremendous stress on the body. All of our organs, including our brains, need water to function properly. When you're dehydrated, your brain chemistry becomes depleted; the neurotransmitters in the brain require water to function. Symptoms include dry skin, brittle bones, muscle cramps, headaches, dark circles around the eyes and hunger, which is actually thirst.

Hydrate adequately by drinking a minimum of half your weight in ounces of filtered water every day. Add a pinch of unprocessed sea salt to your water for additional trace minerals. The sea salt will encourage your body to absorb the water it receives and will help avoid frequent urination.

**Consume wholesome nutrition – eat real food.** An unhealthy diet can be one of the biggest causes of stress on the body. Fueling your body with the nutrients it needs is vital for reducing stress, healing from adrenal fatigue and staying healthy. Stress can actually deplete your body of vital nutrients. Zinc and magnesium are the first minerals to be depleted under stress.

Make sure to include plenty of protein (our bodies require more protein when we're stressed), fruits, vegetables, seeds and nuts. These foods contain stress-reducing vitamins such as C and E, folic acid and B-complex. Snack on some walnuts. According to researchers at Penn State, walnuts help reduce stress and are the healthiest of all nuts – they're high in antioxidants and a good source of omega-3 fats.

Eat mindfully, chew your food thoroughly and sit down during mealtime to thoroughly enjoy your food. Eliminate news, television, loud music, cell phones, computer and stressful conversations during meals (see *Chapter 13*).

**Listen to music.** Research has discovered that listening to music, specifically slow, quiet, classical music, can decrease the amount of the cortisol produced by the body in response to stress. Countless studies have shown music's relaxing effects can be observed on anyone, including newborns.

Music can also help you get "into the zone" when practicing yoga, self-hypnosis or guided imagery; feel energized when exercising and recovering after exercising; dissolve stress; and promote relaxation when you're soaking in the tub. Upbeat music can take your mind off what stresses you and help you feel more optimistic and positive. Music goes a long way toward helping release stress and can even help you reduce your stress over life's little frustrations in the future.

**Take a walk.** Walking leisurely is especially beneficial for reducing cortisol levels, particularly when done outdoors in nature or with a pet. Pet owners who walk their dog have a lower risk of obesity and are more physically active than those without pets.

**Release attachment to control.** You cannot control other people, events or circumstances. Direct your energy into things you can control. Be aware of your emotional state and the fact that you have the choice to change your thoughts and perception.

**Adopt an attitude of gratitude.** Studies report that daily gratitude exercises produce higher levels of energy, optimism, alertness, enthusiasm and determination, and raise serotonin levels.

Make the choice to be grateful. In other words, consciously start and end your day by looking for those things in your life you are most grateful for. Studies have shown that those who are grateful and express gratitude have lower levels of depression and stress.

Being grateful allows you to focus on the positive elements in your life and value the gifts you already have.

Love, appreciation and gratitude have a profound effect on your health by increasing vitality and vigor, boosting immune function and strengthening chemical production. Gratitude reduces stress hormones; lowers blood pressure and feelings of anxiety, guilt and burnout; and increases glucose metabolism.

Every night I pull out my gratitude log and jot down five to ten things, events or people I am grateful for. I also have a gratitude rock on my nightstand. Before I go to sleep each night, I hold this rock and give thanks for the best thing that happened that day. Try it for yourself and experience the positive mental state these small exercises can produce.

**De-clutter.** Clutter will make your life feel more complicated than it needs to be. A clutter-free space is peaceful. Eliminate anything or anyone that is not improving the quality of your life. Manage your to-do list and set boundaries.

**Move your body.** Aside from strengthening your heart and lungs (two organs that can become physically affected from too much stress), exercise is highly beneficial for your mental health too. Exercise will increase the levels of endorphins in your body, which stimulate your immune system and elevate your mood.

Don't overdo it though! Too much exercise is a chronic stressor and adversarial to your fat loss efforts. Participate in an intelligently designed exercise program paired with more relaxing, yin-style activities such as walking, preferably outdoors in nature; Tai chi; Qi gong or restorative yoga. Yoga can reduce stress by signaling to your brain to lower cortisol levels.

Exercise bouts of 30 minutes, but not longer than 60 minutes, appear to have the best stress-reducing benefits. Moderate to vigorous activities reduce stress better than low intensity activity. You must be healthy, nourished with wholesome foods and well-rested with balanced hormones to benefit and recover properly from more intense exercise. Working out too hard, too much and too often without addressing these other important variables compromises your immune system and causes hormonal imbalances.

**Be charitable.** Charitable acts and volunteering have been shown to decrease stress, improve quality of life, enrich sense of purpose and increase lifespan for the giver, while a person who receives, but does not practice charity, doesn't experience the same benefit.

**Relax in the tub.** Schedule time to soak in a relaxing bath with four to six cups of Epsom salts added. The magnesium from the Epsom salts will be absorbed into the skin, aiding in muscle relaxation. Add a few drops of aromatherapy oil, such as lavender. Light candles around the tub. This is one of the most powerful ways to relax and connect with your mind, body and soul.

**Feel positive.** Don't just think positive, *feel* positive. Recall a positive moment or fun time in your life and attempt to re-live it in your mind. Sustain that positive feeling for at least 20 seconds.

**Reduce exposure to electromagnetic stress.** Turn off all communications devices at a set time each night, including your cell phone, iPad, computer, television and fax. Remove electronic devices from your sleeping area.

**Support your digestive system.** The body's second brain is in the gut, which is lined with a network of neurons and neurotransmitters. The gut-brain oversees digestion, absorption and excretion. Prolonged stress can affect the digestive system, causing reduced nutrient absorption and enzymatic output. As a result, blood flow to the gut decreases, which causes a lowered metabolism and digestive dysfunction (see *Chapter 6*).

**Get restful sleep.** During sleep, the stress hormone cortisol is lowered. Sleep deprivation causes cortisol levels to rise. Turn off the lights by 10:00 p.m. According to the National Institutes of Health, the physical body repairs between the hours of 10:00 p.m. and 2:00 a.m., and the mental-emotional-spiritual body repairs between the hours of 2:00 a.m. and 6:00 a.m.

**Enjoy cocoa and cacao.** These may actually help reduce your stress levels. According to a study published in the *Journal of Proteome Research*, eating half an ounce of dark chocolate a day for two weeks reduced levels of stress hormones, catecholamines and cortisol in people feeling highly stressed, and partially corrected other stress-related biochemical imbalances.

Dark chocolate is high in magnesium, the "anti-stress" mineral, and has natural anti-depressant properties, releasing serotonin and stimulating the secretion of endorphins to relieve stress.

However, the health benefits of chocolate apply only to dark chocolate with a cocoa content of at least 70 percent cocoa. Enjoy a hot cup of homemade cocoa by adding one teaspoon of organic cocoa into a heated cup of water. Sweeten it with stevia. Sip, relax and distress.

**Sip on some tea.** Various herbal teas are beneficial for stress, anxiety and exhaustion. Try one of the following teas to experience a calming, relaxing effect and sense of relief from stress: chamomile, ashwagandha, skullcap, Siberian ginseng or passion flower tea.

Research suggests that drinking five or more cups of green tea daily may reduce the incidence of psychological distress by 20 percent!

**Get a pet.** Pets help calm us down. Owning a pet can reduce stress hormones. Most pet owners say companionship, love, company and affection are the main benefits to owning a pet.

**Build strong friendships and loving relationships.** Surround yourself with like-minded people who lift you up and make you feel good. Determine who and what is most important to you, and center your life with those people and items. Resign from negative influences and situations, energy vampires and commitments that are not fulfilling to you.

**Stress–reducing nutrients and herbs:**

| | |
|---|---|
| * Adrenal support | * Magnesium |
| * Ashwagandha | * Omega-3 fatty acids |
| * HCL / Digestive support | * Panax Ginseng |
| * Phosphatidylserine | * Rhodiola |
| * Siberian ginseng | * Vitamin C |
| * Vitamin B complex with pantothenic acid | * Unprocessed sea salt (trace minerals) |

It is important to remember that the body doesn't differentiate between types of stress, and each of us has an individual, unique response to the stressors in our life, some of which is determined by our genetic makeup. However, much of it is within our control if we understand how our perception and choices affect our health. Robert Crayhon, M.S. said, "pleasure is the most important nutrient." Determine what brings you joy and practice it regularly.

## Snooze to lose – sleep for a Hot 'n Healthy Body

Are you having trouble losing body fat, despite the fact that you're eating clean and exercising frequently? Don't underestimate the power of sleep when it comes to losing body fat.

Sleep has a profound impact on the size of your waist and the size of your appetite. Many individuals focus solely on diet and exercise, and fail to consider the importance sleep has on optimal health and losing body fat. Any deep sleep, whether in an eight-hour block or a 30-minute nap, also increases cognitive function and primes our brains to function at a higher level. For optimal health and faster and lasting fat loss, prioritize sleep!

**Let's talk hormones again!** A study in *Endocrine Development* reports that as few as two sleepless nights can damage your metabolism by increasing levels of the hormone ghrelin, stimulating hunger and decreasing levels of the hormone leptin, which tells you to stop munching. When you're sleep-deprived, the ratio between leptin and ghrelin is disrupted, causing you to feel hungrier and eat more food, especially carbohydrates, sugar and junk food.

Research also notes that sleep debt causes insulin resistance and interferes with fat metabolism. Just a few nights of poor sleep can make your cells resistant to insulin, which in turn triggers higher insulin levels and increased body fat. Studies in the *Annals of Internal Medicine* found that after four nights of short sleep the insulin sensitivity of fat cells decreased by 30 percent, and that sleeping less than eight hours a night is counter-productive to fat burning.

Human growth hormone (HGH), a.k.a. the "youth" hormone, is produced naturally in the pituitary gland. HGH is secreted during sleep and vigorous exercise. It helps prevent aging, promote growth in your muscles, tendons and ligaments, boost your immune system and burn fat. Optimal secretion depends on deep, restful sleep for eight hours.

When you're sleep-deprived, you make less HGH and increase the likelihood of increased body fat storage. In addition, just one week of short sleep (five hours) creates a 10-15 percent drop in testosterone.

Sleep deprivation also causes cortisol levels to rise. Normally, cortisol production decreases between midnight and 4:00 a.m. If cortisol levels continually stay elevated, quality sleep and losing stubborn belly fat will never happen. In this sense, managing stress and balancing hormones become a priority so you can get a restful night's sleep and melt the fat away.

Besides disrupting hunger and satiation hormones, poor sleep increases cravings for sugar, carbs and junk food and a greater risk of developing insulin resistance. When you fail to get the required seven to nine hours of sleep, inflammation also increases, and your ability to secrete and regulate hormones diminishes, which accelerates aging and adds inches to your waistline! It's a vicious cycle.

A study in the journal *SLEEP* suggests that the amount of sleep you get has an effect on your gene expression. In other words, getting enough sleep appears to reduce the genetic risk of being overweight or obese, making diet, exercise and other controllable lifestyle factors more effective for fat loss. The less you sleep, the more important genetic factors are in how much body fat you have. The longer you sleep, the greater the influence environmental factors such as meal composition and timing have on obtaining your fat loss goals. When you're constantly deprived of shut-eye, you remain in a state of stress, and the genes that code for that stressful situation relay the message that you need to hold onto calories.

Researchers in Canada found that adding an hour of nightly shut-eye could mean a decrease in more than a pound and a half of fat mass. People who slept six or fewer hours a night gained an average of more than five pounds. On the other hand, those who adjusted their sleep habits to a healthier seven to nine hours per night didn't gain any weight.

*Revolution Solutions* – overcome insomnia

**Create an environment for restful sleep.** As evening approaches, reduce exposure to blue light, which suppresses normal melatonin production. Blue light is a part of the light spectrum that is especially visible during the day, making its appearance a cue to the body to wake up. Televisions, cell phones and computer screens emit blue lights that reduce and limit melatonin production. Use candles, and dim the lights in your home an hour or so before bedtime.

**Sleep in complete darkness**. Make your bedroom pitch black. If there is even the tiniest bit of light in the room it can disrupt your circadian rhythm and your pineal gland's production of melatonin and serotonin. Minimize light in the bathroom too, in case you get up in the middle of the night. Keep the lights off if you go to the bathroom at night because as soon as you turn on that light, you immediately stop production of an important sleep aid, melatonin.

**Avoid the computer and television at least two hours before bedtime**. Working, using the computer and cell phones and texting within two hours of bedtime delay sleep and increase awakenings. Keep the television and your laptop out of the bedroom. If you're accustomed to watching TV or doing work on your laptop in bed, it will be harder for you to relax and get restful sleep.

**Install f.lux, a free program, on your computer** to **reduce blue light emissions.** The program adjusts your computer's color temperature according to the location and time of day. Blue light regulates the secretion of melatonin. http://stereopsis.com/flux

**Meditate.** Just two to five minutes can induce restful sleep. Practice deep belly breathing and yoga postures such as forward folding and legs up the wall.

**Address food sensitivities.** Avoid dairy, sugar, soy, wheat, corn, gluten and omega-6 fats, which cause sleep apnea and disrupted sleep.

**Exercise regularly**. Exercising for at least 30 minutes every day will help you fall asleep. However, exercising too close to bedtime may keep you awake. Sleep is an important component to exercise recovery.

**Avoid caffeine later in the day**. A recent study showed that in some people, caffeine is not metabolized efficiently and they feel the effects long after consuming it. For those individuals, it is best to stay away from caffeine after noon.

**Keep bedroom temperature no higher than 70 degrees F.** Many people keep their homes, and particularly the upstairs bedrooms, too hot.

**Lose weight.** Being overweight increases the risk of sleep apnea, which will prevent a restful nights' sleep.

**Rule out adrenal hypofunction and reactive hypoglycemia.** If you can fall asleep, but are unable to stay asleep, eat a high-protein snack an hour or so before bed, or consume an easily digestible whey protein shake, which will provide your body with L-tryptophan, needed to produce melatonin and serotonin. Avoid grains, processed carbs and sugars that raise blood sugar and inhibit growth hormone release.

**Hydrate during the day**. If you're dehydrated, your body's production of cortisol increases, while melatonin and growth hormone decrease, which will disrupt sleep. Minimize fluid intake within two hours of going to bed. This will reduce the likelihood of needing to get up and go to the bathroom or at least minimize the frequency. If you do need to get up for the bathroom, refrain from turning on lights.

**Take a hot bath, shower or sauna** before bed. Add some Epsom salts to the bath. The magnesium is absorbed through your skin and promotes muscular relaxation. Add a few drops of essential aromatic oils, such as lavender or vanilla, which will induce a state of calm, thereby enhancing sleep.

**Go to bed earlier**. Make sleep a priority and go to bed no later than 10:00 p.m. When you stay up later, particularly after midnight, a disrupted cortisol production pattern occurs. Our bodies, particularly the adrenal glands, do a majority of their recharging or recovering between the hours of 11:00 p.m. and 1:00 a.m. This time frame is also when 80 percent of growth hormone is secreted, and when your gallbladder meridian is most active and releases toxins. If you are awake, the toxins back up into the liver, which secondarily backs up into your entire system and causes further disruption to your health. If you consistently wake up between the 1:00 a.m. and 3:00 a.m., this may indicate liver toxicity or a congested liver, as these are the hours when the liver meridian is most active. Regularly waking between 3:00 a.m. and 5:00 a.m. indicates oxidative stress. If this is the case, your body is in need of antioxidants to combat the free radical damage to your cells that oxidative stress can cause.

**Write in a gratitude journal.** Before bed, log three to five things you're grateful for in your journal.

**Avoid alcohol.** Although alcohol can make you drowsy, the effect is short-lived, and you'll often wake up several hours later unable to fall back asleep. Alcohol keeps you from falling into the deeper stages of sleep, plus it disrupts and inhibits growth hormone production.

**Rule out parasites,** since parasites are more active at night.

**Move loud alarm clocks.** They can be very stressful on your body. If an electric alarm clock must be used, keep it as far away from the bed as possible, preferably at least five feet, because of electro-magnetic fields (EMFs). Electric blankets and plugged in cell phones also emit EMFs. EMF exposure disrupts the pineal gland and the production of melatonin and serotonin, and comes with a host of other negative effects. If you must use a clock, cover it and remove it from view. It will only add to your worry when constantly starring at it... 2:00 a.m....3:00 a.m....4:30 a.m.

**Manage stress.** According to sleep experts, stress is the number one cause of insomnia. Identify your stressors and implement some of the healthy stress-less solutions.

**Test hormones**, including thyroid and adrenals. Insomnia is often a symptom of overtaxed adrenals. Hormonal disruption often occurs during perimenopause, menopause, andropause and high stress lifestyles. These are also cases where individuals experience the most sleeplessness.

**Read something spiritual** to help you relax. Refrain from reading anything stimulating, such as a mystery or suspense novel – this may have the opposite effect.

**Relax with aromatherapy.** Sprinkle a few drops of lavender, sandalwood or vanilla oil on your pillow to induce restful sleep.

**Go to bed and wake up at the same time each day**, even on the weekends. This will help your body to get into a sleep rhythm, making it easier to fall asleep and get up in the morning. Erratic schedules disrupt your body clock.

**Listen to white noise, guided mediation or relaxation CDs.** Some people find the sound of white noise or nature sounds, such as the sounds of ocean waves, very soothing for sleep.

**Wear socks to bed** to avoid waking throughout the night. Your feet have the poorest circulation in the body and will usually feel cold before the rest of the body.

**Try an overnight fast**, which not only boosts your metabolism, it allows your body to shift into a fat burning zone without dieting. Overnight fasting means your last meal of the day is at 6:00 p.m. You forego any late night snacks after dinner and resume eating at breakfast the next morning.

**Add nutritional support** to encourage restful sleep. The first nutrient to consider is magnesium, nature's natural muscle relaxer. Magnesium deficiency is common in 90 percent of the population. Start with 300mg up to 800mg taken 30-60 minutes before bedtime, and determine what dose works best for you. Another option is rubbing magnesium oil or gel behind your knees before retiring each night.

If you are unable to fall asleep, the problem is usually a need for alkaline minerals, and a need to balance the central nervous system (sympathetic-stimulation, parasympathetic-relaxation). For anxiety, consider inositol; the amino acid GABA; Insomnitol; or VHP, a blend of Valerian, Hops and Passion Flower, an excellent herbal tranquilizer without side effects. Be aware that many OTC and prescription medications can affect sleep negatively.

**Consider melatonin** and its precursor, L-tryptophan, or 5-HTP, a precursor to serotonin. If behavioral changes don't work, melatonin may help. Melatonin is a powerful hormone and comes with other redeeming benefits aside from promoting restful sleep. A study published in *Physiology and Behavior* reported that when melatonin is taken before exercise, it is linked to reduced oxidative damage, lower cortisol, improved immune defenses and increased fat burning.

Be aware that melatonin *in excess* can inhibit the thyroid and immune system. Ideally, it is best to increase levels of melatonin naturally with exposure to bright sunlight in the daytime along with full spectrum fluorescent bulbs in the winter, and complete darkness at night. Your bedroom should be completely dark so no light is coming in from the outside. *5-HTP should not be used during pregnancy or lactation, by individuals taking antidepressant drugs or those with cardiovascular disease.* Always discuss melatonin and all other supplementation with your healthcare practitioner prior to use.

## Let's Review the *Revolution Solutions* for Flat Abs

In review of *Chapter 5*, the *Fat Loss Revolution Solutions* to obtaining hot and healthy looking abs must include the following:

* Adhere to the *Fat Loss Revolution* (FLR) eating plan.

* Balance hormones, specifically insulin and cortisol.

* Consider food sensitivities and intolerances and remove those foods from your diet.

* Make it a priority to get seven to nine hours of restful sleep every night.

* Exercise consistently with the FLR workout programs.

* Manage your stressors with some of the FLR stress-less solutions.

* Monitor portions that include protein and fiber from leafy greens, non-starchy vegetables or berries at every meal.

> *Follow the principles in the* Fat Loss Revolution *to diminish bloating, melt your muffin top and attain sexier, flatter abs!*

# CHAPTER 6

## A HAPPY, HEALTHY GUT FOR A HOT 'N HEALTHY BODY

A strong, healthy functioning digestive system is the foundation for optimal health and plays a significant role in your ability to lose body fat. The primary function of the digestive system is to break down and absorb the nutrients from the food we eat into smaller parts so the body can use them to build and nourish cells and provide energy.

Franz Ingelfinger, M.D., a gastroenterologist and late editor of the *New England Journal of Medicine,* estimated that 85 percent of all human illnesses are curable by the body's own healing mechanisms. As the most prominent gastrointestinal physician of his day, he recognized that poor digestion would, in time, undermine every other aspect of health.

The gut is considered your second brain. Over two-thirds of neurotransmitters are made in the gut. Approximately 90 percent of serotonin is manufactured in the gut, not in the brain. If the gut is inflamed or not functioning optimally, production of serotonin and other neurotransmitters that are required to stay healthy will be impaired, and the end result is depression. With one in four American women on prescription drugs for stress, anxiety and depression, addressing gut dysfunction should be prioritized and cannot be overlooked.

In addition to neurotransmitters, 80 percent of the immune system cells line the gastrointestinal tract, creating a protective, impermeable barrier. Damage from unhealthy bacteria, viruses, parasites, alcohol, caffeine, excess sugar, anti-inflammatory drugs, antibiotics and many food substances will activate the immune and stress response mechanisms in the body, which can destroy this protective barrier.

Healthy intestinal bacteria are crucial for optimal health, weight maintenance and a healthy metabolism. Harmful bacteria increase inflammation in the body and make cells less sensitive to insulin. This creates yet another underlying problem that must be addressed to achieve optimal health and permanent fat loss.

**Causes and conditions of harmful bacteria in the gut:**
* Environmental chemicals
* Inflammatory intestinal diseases: IBS, Crohn's disease, colitis, dysbiosis, diverticulitis, leaky gut syndrome and other gastrointestinal conditions
* Lack of HCL (hydrochloric acid)
* Long-term use of antibiotics, NSAIDs or steroid drugs
* Parasites, Candida, H. pylori and other gut pathogens
* Sugar, alcohol, processed foods, conventionally-raised meats and rBGH-laced milk

Your gut can become inflamed from any foreign substance, such as rancid cooking oils, environmental toxins, parasites or foods your body is sensitive to or intolerant of, which increases an inflammatory response. This leads to excess cortisol production, which is directly linked to stubborn lower belly fat and thigh fat, an inflamed brain, depression, dementia and a host of other health conditions.

Food allergies and intolerances often are the main cause of metabolic and gastrointestinal inflammation. Therefore, the easiest and safest mode of healing metabolic and gastrointestinal inflammation is to follow a non-inflammatory diet that excludes trigger foods.

**Obtain proof with lab testing to identify the main triggers:**
* CBC, HbA1C, HLA genetic testing and IgA stool titers
* IgG testing, gluten, casein, egg, legume (soy), environmental allergens and parasites

# The 4R Gut Restoration Program

## Remove – Repair – Restore – Replace

The 4R Program developed by Jeffrey Bland, Ph.D., of the Institute of Functional Medicine, is an extremely effective method to address and heal gut dysfunction and restore and promote gastrointestinal health.

## Step 1 – Remove

* Toxins in food
* Gastric irritants (caffeine, soy, gluten, sugar, alcohol and non-steroidal anti-inflammatory drugs)
* Food allergies, sensitivities, intolerances or reactions
* Chronic low-grade infections in the gut (e.g., yeast, parasites, H. pylori and C. difficile) that can flourish for years without causing noticeable symptoms

## Step 2 – Replace

* Stomach acid (address HCL deficiency)
* Broad-spectrum digestive enzymes

## Step 3 – Restore

* Restore beneficial bacteria with probiotics to re-establish a healthy balance of microflora in the gut.

## Step 4 – Repair

* Provide nutrients to heal the gut wall or lining.
* Support the immune functioning of the gut.

## Step 1 – Remove

Remove all inflammatory items, specifically: gluten, corn, wheat, sugar, polyunsaturated vegetable oils, pasteurized dairy and foods containing trans fats and hydrogenated oils. Avoid conventionally-raised meats and rBGH-laced milk (see *Chapter 4*).

These foods trigger inflammation in your gut lining, causing the healthy, tight junctions in between the cells of the GI tract to loosen. This is known as "leaky gut." A leaky gut allows undigested food particles or other substances such as toxins, microbes, wastes, antigens and pathogens into the bloodstream that don't belong there. This causes gas, bloating, diarrhea, constipation, food sensitivities, skin conditions, depression, fatigue, a compromised immune system and more inflammation. Over time, inflammation in the gut will lead to inflammation in the bones, heart and brain.

**Candida.** Nearly three out of four people suffer from some type of yeast problem (Candida) and have no idea that this is the root cause of their problems. Symptoms may include rashes, bad breath, increased PMS, bloating and brain fog, along with more serious conditions including depression, joint pain, irritable bowel syndrome, depression and even chronic fatigue syndrome. Therefore, another component of step one is ruling out Candida, parasites or other pathogenic bugs that may be contributing to ill health, extra weight gain, bloating and other problems that indicate your body is out of balance.

Adhering to the dietary principles in the *Fat Loss Revolution*, with specific attention to avoiding all sugar, refined grains, dairy and alcohol, will destroy the problematic Candida. Include cultured foods, pau d' arco tea, coconut oil and plenty of garlic, ginger and oregano. A specific supplemental protocol to overcome Candida overgrowth including emulsified oil of oregano and caprylic acid will help destroy the pathogen. This program should be followed for six to eight weeks. Immediately afterward, the focus is directed toward rebuilding the intestinal environment with good bacteria found in cultured foods and supplements, prebiotics and probiotics.

**Parasites.** It has been estimated that 90 percent of humans are walking around with an active intestinal parasite infection. When parasites infect the body, they consume food and absorb the very nutrients you need, leading to vitamin and nutrient deficiencies, draining your energy, producing toxic wastes and eventually destroying your tissues and cells.

Warning signs and symptoms of a parasite infection may include:
* a burning sensation in the stomach
* anemia
* chronic fatigue
* dark circles under the eyes
* diarrhea or constipation
* digestion difficulties
* food and environmental allergies
* inability to gain or lose weight
* itching around the eyes, nose, ears or anus
* joint and muscle aches and pains
* loss of appetite or overeating
* persistent skin problems such as hives, rashes, sores, eczema
* sexual dysfunction
* slower reflexes
* sudden blurred vision
* teeth grinding
* unexplained gas and bloating
* unexplained menstrual problems

Along with eating organic foods, completely avoiding sugar and managing stress, research shows that natural ingredients such as black walnut, oil of oregano, coconut oil bromelain, grapefruit seed, cloves, slippery elm, wormwood and pau d' arco extract and tea can help combat parasites.

Always complete a comprehensive digestive stool analysis (CSDA) to determine the type of parasite and the severity of the infestation.

## Step 2 – Replace

Hydrochloric acid (HCL) is found in the stomach in a diluted form. It acidifies the stomach, acting as a barrier against micro-organisms to prevent infection and is important for digestion of food.

HCL is necessary for protein digestion and the assimilation of B12, folate and 15 minerals. Many people with low stomach acid, hypochlorhydria, or no stomach acid, achlorhydria, often complain of bloating, belching, a feeling of heaviness in the stomach after eating, or feeling full after eating only a small amount of food. Individuals with insufficient stomach acid may experience constipation, while others have diarrhea. And yet some people with little or no stomach acid who experience no symptoms at all.

Research shows that the natural levels of HCL and digestive enzymes decrease due to the aging process, inflammation, stressful lifestyles and abusing our bodies and gastrointestinal tracts through food excesses and chemical use.

As we age, our stomachs make less and less acid. By the time we are 60 years old, our stomach acid is 75 percent lower than when we were 20. In addition, Robert Rakowski, D.C., C.C.N., estimates that 98 percent of the American population is deficient in HCL because of increased stress levels.

Lack of HCL causes carbohydrates to ferment and protein to putrefy in your body. HCL deficiency inhibits your body's ability to break down, absorb and use the food you eat or the supplements you take at the cellular level, creating an environment of malnourishment. If you are not digesting your food properly, your risk of Candida, leaky gut and other health conditions and diseases increases.

Insufficient digestive enzymes and HCL deficiency can contribute to excess body fat, an inability to lose body fat and a host of other symptoms.

A simple remedy for achlohydria and hypochlohydria is to supplement with HCL, *not* over-the-counter antacids or prescription drugs. When you take supplemental betaine hydrochloride combined with digestive enzymes (Digestzymes), you can expect improved digestion and assimilation of protein, amino acids, minerals and other important nutrients. Your energy, strength, endurance and sleep will also improve.

Digestive enzymes are essential to the body's absorption and full utilization of food. They help increase the chemical reactions that break down food in the digestive tract.

Antacids and commonly prescribed drugs for heartburn (e.g., Zantac, Mylanta, Tagamet and Nexium, the "purple" pill) inhibit HCL production and set the stage for later degenerative diseases by interfering with digestion and absorption of minerals, proteins and vitamins. These drugs neutralize stomach acid and reduce or block stomach acid production – exactly what you don't want. Many commercial antacids contain toxic ingredients such as aluminum, artificial colors and sweeteners. Jonathan Wright, M.D., says, "These chemicals disrupt digestion and alter the structure and function of stomach lining cells and cause side effects like headache, diarrhea and abdominal pain."

## Take the HCL test – determine your personal dose

Start with two Digestzyme capsules in the middle of the meal. For the HCL test, all meals must include animal protein. Eat half of your protein and take two capsules.

Notice when a warming sensation develops in the upper abdomen area. If you do not feel a warming sensation in your stomach, at your next meal, increase to three capsules.

Continue to increase by one capsule per meal until you feel a warming sensation. Once you feel a warming sensation, back off by one capsule. This will be your personal dose per meal. For instance, if you feel a warming sensation at five capsules, your dose is four capsules per meal.

The initial optimum dose may be quite high; however, it will decrease over time to a lower maintenance dosage.

*NOTE: Do not take the HCL test if you have a peptic ulcer.*

## Step 3 – Restore

**Prebiotics** are non-digestible food ingredients that nourish and stimulate the growth of beneficial bacterial so they can thrive in the intestinal tract. Basically, prebiotics are food for your flora. Prebiotics may reduce appetite and increase satiety. They help improve insulin sensitivity and reduce visceral fat.

**Probiotics** (from "pro" and "biotia," meaning "for life") are live organisms that reinocculate the gastrointestinal tract with healthy bacteria. When you have adequate beneficial flora, you have a protective barrier against substances that travel through the intestines. A study published in the *European Journal of Clinical Nutrition* found probiotics beneficial for fat loss, specifically belly fat.

**Benefits of probiotics:**
* Boost immune function
* Decrease belly fat
* Encourage healthy gut flora and nutrient absorption
* Improve insulin sensitivity
* Lower cortisol levels
* Prevent and treat vaginal yeast infections and urinary tract infections
* Promote regularity of bowel function
* Protect against harmful bacteria
* Reduce inflammation and the risk of chronic disease
* Relieve constipation and encourage healthy elimination
* Speed up metabolism
* Support weight loss
* Support the digestive system, improving digestion
* Taken during the first trimester of pregnancy, help women lose weight after childbirth
* Favorable for overall health

Healthy probiotic-rich foods include fermented vegetables and natto, yogurt, kefir and sauerkraut, which are naturally fermented and unpasteurized.

There are also foods that do not contain bacteria, but do encourage good bacteria growth. These are known as prebiotics and can be obtained by eating certain foods, including garlic, onions, leeks, jicama, artichokes and the superfood, chlorella.

Prebiotics combined with probiotics (called synbiotics) are more effective at gut modulation than either taken alone.

*Revolution Solutions* **to optimize digestion:**

* Avoid carbonated beverages.

* Avoid eating meals under stressful conditions. Turn off the news or chaotic music while dining; even stressful conversations during mealtime can disrupt digestion.

* Be fully present (mind, body and soul) when eating. Make your mealtime an enjoyable experience.

* Chew your food until it is liquefied before swallowing.

* Consume prebiotics.

* Drink a cup of water with the juice of half a lemon or lime *before* meals.

* Drink plenty of clean, filtered water *away from meals.*

* Drinking water during mealtime dilutes HCL and weakens digestion.

* Eat more fermented foods (sauerkraut, kefir, miso paste, and plain, full fat yogurt with live and active cultures)

* Eliminate toxic foods that your body is intolerant of that wreak havoc on your GI system, specifically gluten, wheat, processed foods, soy and dairy.

* Go for a walk after eating.

* Maintain a healthy weight. Extra weight puts pressure on your abdomen and can encourage acid reflux.

* Take probiotics. *Saccharomyces boulardii* supports the health of the GI tract, protects against intestinal dysbiosis, is effective against Candida overgrowth and prevents Candida from forming.

* Refrain from lying down for two to three hours after eating.

* Rule out parasites or any other intestinal pathogen.

* Supplement with probiotics *at the end of your meal or before bedtime* (not at the same time as HCL or the digestive enzymes).

* Take Digestzymes or Betaine Plus HP *in the middle of the meal.* Drink only enough water to wash them down.

* Take one to three teaspoons of apple cider vinegar in water 15 minutes before meals for optimal absorption of vitamins and minerals from your food. (This is not recommended for those with ulcers.)

## Step 4 – Repair

**Nutrients to heal the gut** – these items will vary per individual:

* Aloe vera

* Curcumin

* Digestive enzymes – Digestzymes

* Emulsified oil of oregano (Biotics ADP)

* Essential fatty acids

* Quercetin

* Methionine

* N-acetyl-cysteine (NAC)

* L-Glutamine powder

* Zinc

* Low-antigen medical foods (Nutriclear, Mediclear, Protoclear)

* Prebiotics – inulin, oligofructose, fructooligosaccharides (FOS), galactooligosaccharides (GOS)

* Probiotics – *Bifidobacteria, Lactobacillus GG, Lactobacillus rhamnosus, Saccharomyces boulardii*

* Teas: Pau 'd Arco, Dandelion, Slippery Elm, Ginger, Peppermint

*A Happy Gut Equals a Happy, Healthy Person.*

# Chapter 7

## THE GOOD, THE BAD AND THE DEADLY AND THEIR IMPACTS ON A HOT 'N HEALTHY BODY

### Frankenfoods, Frankenfats and Obesogens – Oh, No!

**F**rankenfood is food that has been engineered, processed or genetically modified, or that contains genetically modified organisms (GMOs). Frankenfoods represent 98 percent of the food produced and consumed by Americans – a scary fact. Fast foods, cookies, chips and crackers, cereals and products with high fructose corn syrup are just a few examples of Frankenfoods. Ninety percent or more of all corn, soybeans, alfalfa, rice, canola and cottonseed oils, and sugar beets grown in the U.S. are genetically modified! Often found in processed foods, GMOs are also found in fruits and vegetables, and in alarming quantities in animal feed.

**Frankenfats** are fake, synthetic, man-made fats that interfere with proper metabolism, promote inflammation and oxidize easily. They are plastic-like and have an endless shelf life. Instead of promoting health, frankenfats elevate risk of heart disease, diabetes and cancer, and increase body fat, suppress the thyroid and accelerate aging. Frankenfats include hydrogenated oil, partially hydrogenated oil, soybean oil, cottonseed oil, canola oil, vegetable oils, fake butter substitutes, margarine and all cooking sprays. Frankenfats are hiding in breads, cakes, cookies, crackers, salad dressings and frozen dinners.

Consuming frankenfats and frankenfoods triggers immune dysfunction and leads to serious health problems.

**Real food** is nutrient-rich, wholesome and free of synthetic hormones, antibiotics, chemicals and GMOs. Real food is produced with integrity, using clean and fair farming practices, developed and harvested by ecologically and socially responsible farmers. Sadly, this represents less than two percent of the total U.S. agriculture.

## Go Organic for a Hot 'n Healthy Body at Any Age

Every day the average American is exposed to 10 to 13 different pesticides through food, beverages and drinking water. Nine of the most common pesticides cause hormone disruption, which has been linked to weight gain. For these reasons alone, it is extremely important to choose to eat wholesome, nutrient-rich foods from organic sources versus conventionally-grown or raised foods.

Organic foods are approximately 40 times more nutritious than commercially farmed foods. Organic fruits and vegetables have up to 40 percent more antioxidants than non-organically grown produce, and on average 180 times lower pesticide content than conventional products. Consuming organic foods can reduce dietary pesticide ingestion by 97 percent!

Fifty years ago, all of our foods were considered organic. An organic food is one that is grown *without* the use of pesticides, herbicides, fungicides, synthetic fertilizers, sewage sludge, genetically modified organisms or ionizing radiation. Organic meat, poultry, eggs and dairy products are produced from animals that are not fed antibiotics, chemicals or synthetic growth hormones.

Organic cattle are those that feed in an organic pasture primarily on grass, hay and legumes void of chemicals, pesticides and fertilizers. These animals are not fed anything containing genetically modified crops, growth hormones, plastic pellets, urea, manure or animal by-products.

Paul Chek, founder of the C.H.E.K Institute and author of *Eat, Move and Be Healthy*, says, "When you choose to eat organic foods, you usually need about 30 percent less food to reach a sense of satiety because the nutrient levels are so much higher that satiety is achieved sooner."

## Grass–fed beef versus grain– or corn–fed beef

### Grass–fed beef – just the facts:

* One of the richest sources of complete protein
* Higher in B vitamins, potassium, selenium, magnesium and zinc
* Ten times higher in beta-carotene
* 60 percent higher in omega-3 fats
* Five times higher in CLA, an important fat for immunity, managing cortisol and visceral fat
* 49 percent lower content of saturated fat
* Zero trans fats
* Four times higher in vitamin E
* Decreased risk of E.coli
* 40 percent decrease in greenhouse gases

Always choose organic, grass-fed and free-range over non-organic and grain-fed, soy-fed and corn-fed when it comes to meats, eggs and dairy products. Animals fed on a diet of grain, soy or corn have a higher fat content, and toxins are stored in the fat. A study in the *International Journal of Obesity* found that the use of hormones in commercial factory meat production could be a possible contributor to the obesity epidemic.

Organic livestock must have access to the outdoors and cannot be given antibiotics or growth hormones. If organic meats are not available, the next best choice is grass-fed, free-range meats. If your budget does not allow you to purchase organic meats and poultry, it is best to reduce your consumption of non-organic sources of animal protein.

If the list of ingredients doesn't include the word "organic" in front of each and every word, *Buyer Beware*. Buy only products that are labeled certified organic to dramatically reduce your exposure to pesticides, hormones and antibiotics, which are used on nearly all GE crops. Products labeled as "USDA 100% organic" must contain *only* organic materials. Products labeled simply "USDA organic" must contain at least 95 percent organic ingredients, whereas the label "made with organic ingredients" can contain anywhere between 70 to 95 percent organic ingredients.

Familiarize yourself with the Environmental Working Group (EWG) Shopper's Guide to Pesticides in Produce. The EWG is a nonprofit organization that examines pesticide levels in commercially grown produce. The EWG shopper's guide reveals which fruits and vegetables are lowest – the "Clean 15" – and highest – the "Dirty Dozen" – in pesticide residues so you'll know which ones you should always buy as organic (see *Resources*).

**The "Dirty Dozen"** (listed in order of highest to lowest pesticides) are apples, celery, strawberries, peaches, spinach, nectarines, grapes, sweet bell pepper, potato, blueberries, lettuce, kale and collards. It is strongly recommended, whenever possible, to purchase the Dirty Dozen fruits and vegetables organically.

**The "Clean 15"** (listed in order from the cleanest to the least clean) are onions, sweet corn, pineapple, avocado, asparagus, sweet peas, mangoes, eggplant, cantaloupe, kiwi, cabbage, watermelon, sweet potatoes, grapefruit and mushrooms.

> *Just because something is labeled organic or gluten-free doesn't make it a healthy food.*
>
> *An organic, gluten-free cookie loaded with sugar and rice flour may have fewer pesticides, but it's still junk food and will create an insulin spike.*

**PLU Codes**

There are unique codes for organic, conventionally grown and genetically modified food items. PLU codes have been used by supermarkets since 1990 to make check-out and inventory control easier, faster and more accurate.

When shopping for fruits and vegetables, you'll notice a PLU code on the sticker, which is usually four digits. The numbers on the sticker indicate if the item is genetically modified, conventional or organic.

A fifth digit may be prefixed to the code to indicate whether the fruit or vegetable is organic (prefixed by the numeral 9), or GM (prefixed by an 8).

Being able to recognize PLU codes can be helpful in your decision to purchase fruits and vegetables.

* **Conventional** – Grown with chemicals and pesticides. The PLU code consists of four numbers.
* **GM** – Genetically modified. The PLU code consists of five numbers beginning with the number 8.
* **Organic** – The five-digit PLU code begins with the number 9.

Sticker examples:
* A conventionally grown apple would be 4021
* A genetically engineered (GE) or modified (GMO) apple would be 84021
* An organic apple would be 94021

Processed foods and most packaged foods are genetically engineered foods that don't carry PLU codes. Ingredients in processed foods – specifically corn, canola oil and soy – are genetically engineered. To avoid GE foods, a great place to start is to eliminate all of the corn, canola oil and soy in your diet and become an avid label reader.

**Avoid the nine primary GE crops:**

* Soy
* Corn
* Canola oil
* Sugar from sugar beets
* Some varieties of zucchini
* Cottonseed
* Hawaiian papaya
* Alfalfa
* Crookneck squash

**Other items that may contain GM ingredients:**

* Infant formula
* Peanut butter
* Protein powder
* Fried foods

* Mayonnaise
* Ice cream
* Frozen yogurt
* Candy and gum

* Beer and alcohol
* Salad dressing
* Bread
* Cereals

* Soy products
* Chips
* Veggie burgers
* Tofu

* Crackers
* Cookies
* Chocolate
* Pasta

* Baking powder
* Tomato sauce
* Margarine
* Hamburgers and hot dogs

The Institute for Responsible Technology has put together a non-GMO shopping guide that can be found by visiting their website, http://www.nongmoshoppingguide.com.

> *One must become educated on how to purchase USDA organic to avoid GMOs and GE food items.*

## Obesogens and Their Impact on Fat Loss

Endocrine-disrupting chemicals (EDCs) are known as obesogens. Obesogens mimic or alter the effects of hormones in the body and often target the estrogen receptors.

These chemicals cause damage to tissue that disrupts insulin sensitivity and glucose balance, accelerates aging, causes infertility, creates brain dysfunction and disturbs the weight regulating hormone, leptin. Additionally, obesogen exposure damages the mitochondria, the place where fat is burned for energy. High blood levels of chlorinated pesticides in adults adversely affect the rate of thermogenesis, your personal thermostat for burning body fat.

Chemical exposure can manifest itself in a wide variety of symptoms, including digestive problems, recurrent Candida, allergies, fatigue, skin problems and even cancer. Furthermore, obesogens inhibit the thyroid, accelerate puberty, increase estrogen, decrease testosterone and lead to sexual dysfunction.

Obesogens play a major role in excess fat storage. They appear to interfere with the body's natural weight-control mechanism, resulting in an increased appetite, a lowered metabolism and a reduced initiative and motivation to participate in physical activity.

Obesogens affects men, women, children and animals. Pregnant women, children and adolescents are especially sensitive to obesogens and should be particularly cautious. Long-term exposure to obesogens alters the function of our hormonal environment, leading to detrimental health outcomes. Obesogens have been linked to hormone-sensitive cancers including endometrial, ovarian, breast and prostate cancer.

**Common obesogens found in the environment, our food and consumer products:**

* Perfluorooctanoic acid (PFOA), a grease-proofing agent used in numerous products from microwave popcorn bags to pizza box liners and other food containers. PFOA is detected in the blood of people around the globe, but is detected at up to 100 times higher concentrations in people living near industrially polluted areas.

* Dioxins, xenoestrogens, pesticides, DDE, DDT

* Heavy metals that act as "metalloestrogens," including cadmium, lead, mercury, aluminum, copper, tin, nickel and others.

* Parabens, which are found in soaps, lotions, shampoos, cosmetics, antiperspirants and deodorants, shaving gel, sunscreens, pharmaceutical drugs and food additives. Parabens can affect your body much like estrogen, which can lead to decreased muscle mass, extra fat storage and male gynecomastia.

* Triclosan, a chlorinated, aromatic compound used as a synthetic broad-spectrum antimicrobial agent found in antibacterial soaps. Triclosan is linked with liver toxicity.

* Organ chlorines, which are used to manufacture pesticides. They're also used in dry cleaning, the bleaching of feminine-hygiene products and in manufacturing plastic.

* Phthalates, which are used as plasticizers to make plastics more pliable. Phthalates are found in cosmetics, plastic toys, some liquid soaps, adhesives, time-released pharmaceuticals, baby lotion and powder, perfumes, deodorizers, air fresheners, hair spray and food packaging.

* Bisphenol-A (BPA) and bisphenol-S (BPS), petroleum-based chemicals that are ingredients in polycarbonate plastics often found in plastic water bottles, baby bottles, receipt and thermal paper, PVC water lines, canned food and soda can liners, dental sealants and many other products. Bisphenol has over 40 potential adverse health effects and contributes to excess mid-section weight gain.

* PCBs found in fish taken from contaminated waters.

* Tributylin, a chemical used in boat paint and plastic food wrap, and as a fungicide on crops, that has been found to leach into food.

* Obesogens are also commonly found in laundry detergents, nail polish and nail polish remover.

The human body is bombarded with these harmful chemicals every day. This creates a burden on the liver, weakens the immune system and disrupts the delicate balance of hormones.

One of my mentors and teachers, Harry Eidenier, Jr., Ph.D., a food scientist and bio-chemist, said, "We are swimming in a sea of estrogen." We must do what we can to eliminate our exposure to these toxic obesogens as much as possible.

The key to avoiding and limiting exposure to these toxic chemicals starts with awareness. The *Revolution Solution* is to live a lifestyle that minimizes exposure to obesogens and detoxifies these harmful chemicals. Eliminate toxic products and replace them with healthier options when possible. Support through restoring hormone balance, detoxifying, and supporting the immune system will work toward protecting our bodies from these harmful hormone-disrupting chemicals.

***Revolution Solutions* to protect yourself from obesogens:**

* Avoid exposure and eliminate use of the following products:
  * All soy products
  * Non-organic coffee and tea
  * Styrofoam products
  * Anything that has the word "fragrance" on it. Instead, use essential oils.

* Many deodorants and antiperspirants contain parabens and aluminum. Instead, try a pinch of baking soda mixed with water or a small amount of vinegar for a natural deodorant.

* Be aware of noxious gas that comes from copiers and printers, new carpets and fiberboards.

* Become a detective-style label reader.

* Buy only organic, hormone-free animal products (eggs, poultry, meats and dairy).

* Always opt for wild salmon over farmed salmon. Most fish farms feed their fish soy and grains, and fish are given antibiotics and other drugs. The majority of farm-raised fish are contaminated with pesticides, PCBs, dioxins and other industrial chemical residues.

* Include more chlorophyll and organic green tea in your diet. The EGCG found in green tea prevents damage from toxic PCBs.

* Drink plenty of filtered water to flush toxins out of the body.

* Dryer sheets, fabric softeners and detergents disburse petrochemicals right onto your skin. Use laundry detergent that is void of chemicals. Try using white vinegar and baking soda as your laundry detergent and household cleaning agent.

* Prioritize the health of your gut (see *Chapter 6*).

* Eat full fat, organic yogurt that contains live and active cultures or other food containing probiotics to encourage healthy intestinal flora.

* Eat locally-grown, organic foods whenever possible.

* If you use topical hormone (progesterone, testosterone) creams, opt for paraben-free creams.

* Install a high-quality reverse-osmosis water filter in your home. Purchase water filters for drinking, showering and bathing water. Fluoride, arsenic, chlorine, lead and even chemical and pharmaceutical runoffs found in unfiltered water are just a few disruptors our bodies would rather do without.

* Look for personal care and household cleaning products that are chemical-free.

* Reduce the use of canned foods and canned beverages.

* Supplemental calcium D-glucarate, diindolylmethane (DIM) crysin and indol-3-carbinol can reverse and eliminate the synthetic estrogen in our bodies.

* Use glass or ceramic containers to store your food and beverages.

* Wash your hands after handling thermal paper receipts and money.

* If you use plastics, only use those with the codes 1, 2, or 5.

## Crap That Makes You Fat, Sick and Just Plain Miserable

Many individuals are completely unaware that certain food items can be the reason they are fat, sick and just plain miserable. Numerous food items contain additives and chemicals, specifically processed, packaged and fast foods. Eighty percent of the average American diet is from processed, packaged and fast foods. That equates to approximately 12 pounds of additives and chemicals eaten annually! These ingredients are harmful and cause numerous adverse health conditions and complaints.

It is extremely important that you habitually read the list of ingredients on all products. Become familiar with, and avoid the following items or any item that contains the following ingredients:

* Grains, wheat and gluten
* High-fructose corn syrup
* Sugar
* MSG
* Processed soy
* Dyes and food colorings
* Pasteurized dairy
* Vegetable oils (PUFAs)
* Artificial sweeteners
* Frankenfats
* GMOs
* Sodium chloride

## Grains, wheat and gluten

The USDA dietary guidelines advise that people eat several servings of whole grains every day, despite the fact that there is significant evidence suggesting that cereal grains are less than optimal foods for humans. The human genetic makeup and physiology may not be fully adapted to high levels of cereal grain consumption.

Grains, specifically wheat, cause a reaction in the intestines that sets off various symptoms. The ultimate effect of this hidden wear and tear is the slow destruction of the healthy mucosa, or lining tissue, of the small intestine, causing gut permeability, leaky gut syndrome, nutrient deficiencies and an auto-immune response that's similar to an allergic reaction.

Grains, including sprouted wheat and wheat grass, contain anti-nutrients such as gluten, lectins, enzyme inhibitors, mineral binding phytates and oxalates that spike insulin, disrupt normal gut physiology and inhibit weight loss. Lectins, phytates and other anti-nutrients bind with tissues and intestinal cells, interfere with nutrient absorption, and are intrinsically inflammatory and hormone-disruptive substances with a laundry list of adverse health effects. Lectins may cause leptin resistance too (see *Chapter 2*).

Regular consumption of anti-nutrients leads to an inability to absorb minerals, chronic inflammation, autoimmune disease, leaky gut and other health problems.

Foods with high concentrations of lectins include: grains (especially wheat), seeds and nuts, beans and legumes (especially soy), dairy and nightshades (potatoes, tomatoes, eggplant), all of which may be harmful if consumed in excess or uncooked or improperly cooked form. White rice, but not brown rice, is naturally free of the potent anti-nutrients like gluten found in grains such as wheat and barley.

Some traditional cultures consume grains and can tolerate them due to preparation methods such as soaking, sprouting and fermentation, which reduce the anti-nutrients and deactivate the enzyme inhibitors making the grains easier to digest. Even though these methods of preparation improve the nutrient profile, soaking, sprouting and fermenting do not eliminate the anti-nutrients or insulin spike that grains cause. It still does not mean that grains are healthy or that we need to or should consume them.

Conditions and symptoms of sensitivity or intolerance to wheat, grains and gluten may include any of the following:

| | |
|---|---|
| * Bloating and gas | * Candida |
| * Crohn's disease | * Diverticulitis |
| * Diarrhea or constipation | * Brain fog |
| * Elevated blood sugar | * Weight gain and obesity |
| * Excess belly fat | * Autism |
| * Gastrointestinal cancers | * Thyroid disease |
| * Increased belly fat | * Water retention |
| * Insulin and leptin resistance | * Altered gut flora |
| * Nasal and throat mucous | * Joint pain |
| * Risk of type 1 and 2 diabetes | * Brain disorders |
| * Skin rashes, acne | * Inflammation |

Literally hundreds of other adverse health complaints are caused by wheat and gluten. In severe cases, as with celiac disease, there can be seizures, psychosis, violent behavior and self-withdrawal. Most doctors dismiss gluten sensitivity if you don't have a diagnosis of celiac disease.

Scientific literature shows that grain consumption is linked to several health problems. People can be gluten-sensitive without having celiac disease or gluten antibodies and still have inflammation and many other symptoms. Wheat and gluten consumption have been associated with at least 160 health conditions. Even more astonishing is a review in the *New England Journal of Medicine* that listed 55 diseases caused by gluten. Gluten affects almost everyone negatively. Some adverse effects are quite evident; however, many effects are sub-clinical and do not show up for years.

A non-gluten chemical in wheat contains a lectin known as wheat germ agglutinin (WGA) is essentially responsible for many of wheat's hard to diagnose, ill effects and causes damage to bodily tissues. WGA is found in highest concentrations in whole wheat. A single, one-ounce slice of wheat bread contains approximately 500 micrograms of WGA.

Wheat and all processed grains negatively affect insulin levels, raising blood glucose higher than many other foods – higher than six teaspoons of sugar, a Milky Way bar or a Snickers bar.

Gluten intolerance is severely misdiagnosed or undetected because the reaction can appear 12-24 hours after eating gluten. One estimate says that 97 percent of all sufferers don't even know they're intolerant to gluten since most doctors are unfamiliar with it. Gluten intolerance causes multiple nutritional deficiencies and inhibits absorption of many vitamins, minerals and other nutrients.

Gluten is a protein found in the endosperm of grains, especially wheat, rye, spelt and barley. It constitutes about 80 percent of the proteins in wheat, and is composed of the proteins gliadin and glutenin. Gliadin has appetite stimulating effects, causing people to eat approximately 400 more calories a day! Gliadin also binds onto the brain's opiate receptor, making wheat (gluten) a highly addictive substance!

Gluten is purposefully used as an ingredient in some products because it encourages a stronger appetite and non-stop hunger for that item by increasing ghrelin, the "I-want-more-food" hormone. As a result, cravings and an insatiable appetite develop for more of the manufacturer's product.

Gluten also interferes with the hormone leptin, which sends a message to your brain that you're full and signals fat fat to break down. Certain grains cause opiate-like activity in the brain. Both gluten (grain) and casein (milk) contain opiod exorphins. Exorphins are substances that come from outside (exogenous) sources that act similar to drugs such as morphine. Consequently, the exorphins found in gluten causes gluten to be highly addictive, especially for people who are genetically unable to tolerate gluten, which is the majority of people. In effect, this comfort food becomes a toxin in their bodies.

Gluten provides elasticity to dough, which gives breads and bagels their chewiness. Gluten is also used as a food additive in the form of a flavoring, stabilizing or thickening agent, often hidden as dextrin, maltodextrin and dextrose, frequently found in ice cream, soy sauce, ketchup, beer and many other items.

Grain products are high in *insoluble fiber* (fiber that does not dissolve in water). Even though whole grains are recommended by some for healthy digestion, insoluble fiber should not be eaten in excess. Fruits and vegetables contain heart-healthy *soluble* fiber that encourages beneficial gut flora.

William Davis, M.D., cardiologist and author of *Wheat Belly*, explains how today's wheat has been transformed into a nutritionally weakened hybrid that contains 10 times more gluten than the wheat of 50 years ago and is the cause for excess belly fat and the obesity epidemic. Wheat contains amylopectin A, which is more efficiently converted to blood sugar than most other carbohydrates, including table sugar. In fact, two slices of whole wheat bread increase blood sugar levels higher than a candy bar does. Dr. Davis confirms that eliminating wheat from our diets will prevent fat storage, shrink unsightly bulges and reverse a myriad of health problems.

Once you completely remove wheat, grains, gluten and all processed flour-based foods from your diet you will look younger and feel so much better. Bloating, headaches and pain often disappear, and as a bonus you will lose that stubborn belly fat.

The choice to go gluten-free means avoiding breakfast cereals, pasta-based dishes, sandwiches, bagels and processed, packaged foods. Gluten is in every grain except quinoa, millet, amaranth, rice and buckwheat.

Whole wheat, multi-grain breads, cookies, muffins and the like that are labeled gluten-free typically replace wheat with potato starch, tapioca starch, sorghum, rice (flour) starch and corn (flour) starch, which are quickly metabolized into sugar.

Yes, these substitutions are gluten-free; however, the caveat is that these ingredients raise blood sugar higher than whole wheat, which will increase your risk of diabetes and add inches to your waistline, thereby inhibiting fat loss.

The majority of gluten-free products are processed junk food designed with clever marketing designs. In reality, these items are unhealthy and usually contain a high content of sugar, salt, fat and carbohydrates (due to their gluten substitutes), along with low levels of essential nutrients. Instead, look for ingredients like ground almonds and other nuts, coconut flour and ground flaxseed that do not cause blood sugar to skyrocket or trigger any other adverse health conditions.

Beware of hidden sources of gluten unexpectedly found in soy sauce, mustard, beer, salad dressings, frozen dinners, pickles, chips and even OTC medications. Words like graham, spelt, couscous, bulgur, kamut, semolina, and MSG may signal the presence of gluten.

> Gluten–free does not automatically qualify that food as a healthier option. Become a dedicated label reader and learn to recognize hidden sources of gluten. Don't be fooled just because an item is labeled "gluten–free."

## Sugar

Have you ever been plagued by a hard-to-diagnose health problem? You intuitively know something is wrong, but your doctor can't seem to figure out what's causing your health problem. On top of that you cannot seem to lose weight, no matter how hard you try, you feel depressed, can't sleep, feel sluggish, lack mental focus and have lost your libido. Could the culprit be sugar? Absolutely!

Sugar is a toxin that is more addictive than cocaine. It is especially harmful to your liver and other organs. Prolonged consumption has devastating effects on the body.

Consuming sugar comes with consequences: damages skin collagen; promotes wrinkles; increases your appetite; causes joint degeneration, food allergies, ADHD and other behavior disorders; stimulates cholesterol synthesis and inhibits fat loss. It's the perfect fuel source for yeast, fungus and cancer.

Sugar is a mood moderator that has a profound influence on brain function *and* your waistline. Consuming sugar creates advanced glycation end products (AGEs) that promote inflammation and accelerate aging. When you overindulge in sugar, your body releases excess amounts of insulin, which in turn causes a drop in blood sugar, also known as hypoglycemia. This crash leads to eating more calories than necessary, resulting in excess body fat and a host of other health problems.

The average American consumes 175 pounds of sugar per year – that averages to 46 teaspoons per day! Sugar intake depletes B vitamins, calcium and magnesium from the body, and interferes with the ability to break down estrogen. For every molecule of sugar ingested, the body uses 54 molecules of magnesium to process it. The liver needs magnesium and B vitamins, particularly B6, in order to detoxify estrogens.

Sugar-free foods are not any better. They're usually loaded with unhealthy vegetable oils, genetically modified ingredients, chemical preservatives, refined grains and artificial sweeteners, all of which contribute to increased cravings and gastrointestinal distress from the sugar alcohols and inhibit fat loss.

Hidden sources of sugar include granola bars, yogurt, tomato sauce, chewing gum, cereal, bread, bagels, juice, milk, salad dressing, sports drinks, low-fat and non-fat items, flavored coffee creamers, canned fruits and soups, spaghetti sauce, peanut butter, infant formula and ketchup.

Sugar is often disguised in processed and packaged foods, such as evaporated cane juice, corn syrup, barley malt, brown rice syrup and any item that ends with –ose. Opt for healthier alternatives such as stevia or xylitol.

> *Sugar is a poison for health, vitality, longevity and fat loss. Consuming sugary foods (corn, rice, candy, pasta, bagels, breads, muffins, soda and fruit juice) sends a hormonal message to your body that says, "I'm going to store more fat"!*

## Homogenized, pasteurized dairy *does not* do a body good

Pasteurized, homogenized milk contains assorted drugs, antibiotics, pesticides from treated grains, bacteria from infected animals, viral pathogens, genetically altered growth hormones, rBGH, and other xenohormones, chemicals that mimic hormones.

Are you aware that one cup of milk contains over 100 pesticides? Aside from the numerous health problems associated with consumption of milk and dairy, including allergies, osteoporosis, autoimmune, diabetes, and ovarian and prostate cancer, researchers have found that milk causes significant insulin secretion. In fact, milk and milk products stimulate as much insulin secretion as whole wheat.

Some individuals opt for fat-free or low-fat milk thinking they are using healthier versions of milk. Fat-free and low fat milk contains slime powdered milk, which oxidizes cholesterol, leading to arterial damage. In addition, fat-free and low-fat milk are missing CLA, a healthy fat, and are void of fat-soluble vitamins.

Seventy-five percent of the world is lactose intolerant, lacking the lactase enzyme and causing great digestive distress. People with many different health complaints, including those suffering with constipation, bloating, digestive dysfunction, sinus problems and ear infections, notice a significant improvement when they completely avoid milk and dairy.

The U.S. leads the world in dairy consumption and has the highest incidence of osteoporosis and hip fractures. Milk actually leaches calcium from your body and encourages the growth of cancer cells. There is no scientific evidence that consumption of dairy products prevents bone loss. In fact, milk and dairy can actually increase your risk of osteoporosis. A Harvard Nurse's Health study found that those who drank two or more glasses of milk daily suffered more hip fractures than those who drank one cup or less.

According to the Weston A. Price Foundation: "Pasteurization destroys enzymes; diminishes vitamin content; denatures fragile milk proteins; destroys vitamins C, B-12 and B-6; kills beneficial bacteria; promotes pathogens and is associated with allergies, increased tooth decay, colic in infants, growth problems in children, osteoporosis, arthritis, heart disease and cancer. Calves fed pasteurized milk do poorly and many die before maturity. Raw milk sours naturally, but pasteurized milk turns putrid; processors must remove slime and pus from pasteurized milk by a process of centrifugal clarification."

If you're concerned about calcium intake for prevention of bone loss, rest assured – green leafy vegetables are the best source of calcium on the planet! Kale and other brassica greens such as collards, turnips, mustard, and bok choy can be substantial dietary sources of calcium for your diet.

> *Get calcium from broccoli, dandelion greens, kale and other dark leafy greens, sea vegetables and seaweeds, sardines, hazelnuts, almonds, sesame and various nuts and seeds.*

**Examples of the calcium content for brassica vegetables:**
* Collard greens, cooked, 1 cup – 357 mg
* Turnip greens, cooked, 1 cup – 249 mg
* Kale, cooked, 1 cup – 179 mg
* Bok choy, cooked, 1 cup – 158 mg
* Mustard greens, cooked, 1 cup – 152 mg
* Broccoli, cooked, 1 cup – 94 mg

## Corn syrup and high–fructose corn syrup (HFCS)

HFCS are highly processed liquid sugars produced from genetically modified (GM) corn extracted with the chemical solvent glutaraldehyde and frequently contaminated with mercury. HFCS is the number one source of calories for most Americans and leads to excess fat accumulation, thyroid dysfunction, impaired memory, metabolic syndrome and numerous other health problems.

You'll find high-fructose corn syrup in thousands of products, especially in processed foods, fruit drinks, fast food, sodas, syrup that goes into your latte from coffee houses, infant formula, chewing gum, baked goods and many other foods you'd never even imagine. It's in practically all packaged foods.

HFCS is extremely toxic to your liver; increases inflammation, LDL cholesterol and oxidative stress; and creates an aggressive insulin response, thus contributing to type 2 diabetes and increased fat storage. It also causes leptin resistance, further contributing to excess body fat and adverse health conditions.

When too much fructose enters the liver, the liver is unable to process the fructose fast enough for the body to use as sugar. As a result, the body starts making fat cells from fructose and sending them off into the bloodstream as triglycerides.

When you consume foods and beverages that contain fructose, your body stops burning fat, your metabolism slows down, and your liver rapidly converts excess fructose into fat. Consuming fructose turns off your body's ability to control appetite.

A study published in the *Journal of the American College of Nutrition* found that fructose may alter the body's balance of magnesium, leading to increased bone loss. In another study at the University of California, Los Angeles (UCLA), researchers found that pancreatic cancer cells use fructose to divide and multiply. Fructose is basically a superfood for cancer cells.

And yet another study out of UCLA found that consuming HFCS destroys memory, slows mental function and deteriorates brain performance.

Agave has a similar effect as high-fructose corn syrup triggering insulin secretion, which signals your body to accumulate fat. High-fructose corn syrup is 45 percent glucose and 55 percent fructose, and agave is 10 percent glucose and 90 percent fructose.

When you consume sizeable amounts of this type of fructose, it is processed directly by the liver, which increases triglyceride levels; triggers an aggressive insulin response; and causes fatty liver, increased hunger and many other health problems.

Yes, fruits contain fructose, but fruits are also full of fiber and nutrients. The level of fructose is comparatively insignificant, and a lean individual is capable of handling natural fructose from fruits *in limited amounts.* However, if you currently are not at a desirable body composition, remember that any type of excessive fructose consumption will inhibit fat loss.

Fructose and glucose are different molecularly and processed very differently in the body. Glucose is metabolized in the bloodstream rapidly, while fructose is mainly processed in the liver.

Fortunately, there are natural substances that help minimize the damaging effects from consumption of high-fructose corn syrup, including:

* Resveratrol         * Ginger              * Spirulina
* Astaxanthin         * Coconut water       * Chorella
* Garlic              * Omega-3- fatty acids

---

*Bottom line – Avoid all products containing artificial sweeteners, high fructose corn syrup and agave.*

## Artificial sweeteners

Aspartame, sucralose, saccharin, NutraSweet, Splenda, acesulfame-K, Sweet 'N Low, Equal ... To avoid artificial sweeteners, you must become an avid label reader and always read the list of ingredients.

Aspartame is the technical name for the brand names NutraSweet, Sweet 'N Low, Equal and Spoonful. Aspartame is an artificial chemical sweetener consisting of 50 percent phenylalanine, 40 percent aspartic acid and 10 percent methanol. It stimulates the neurons in your brain so drastically that they burn out and cease to function. Aspartame accounts for as many as 75 percent of adverse reactions to food additives reported to the *Food and Drug Administration.*

Aspartame is a known carcinogenic that may cause cancer and neurological problems. The ingredient acesulfame potassium is just another name for aspartame. Acesulfame K is a derivative of acetoacetic acid, another toxin, and contains methylene chloride, a carcinogen.

NutraSweet is in over 8,000 foods, including desserts, gelatins, breath mints, low-calorie foods, sugar-free fruit drinks, sugar-free gum, children's vitamins, wine coolers, flavored bottled waters, cereals, cold remedies and other medications, some protein powders, and of course, diet sodas.

Splenda, another artificial sweetener, contains three molecules of chlorine. Splenda is a carcinogen that shrinks the thymus gland, enlarges the liver and kidneys and triggers weight gain. Splenda also kills friendly intestinal bacteria and inhibits absorption of iodine in the thyroid gland.

Researchers have repeatedly found that artificial sweeteners intensify cravings for sugar and carbohydrates, inhibit fat loss and actually trigger weight gain. One University of Texas study found that consuming just one 12 ounce diet soda a day increases a person's risk of metabolic syndrome, heart disease and obesity by 40 percent!

In a 2008 Purdue study, animals that were fed artificial sweeteners ate more food and put on 14 percent more body fat.

A clear link has been established between the consumption of artificial sweeteners and the increased risk of gaining weight. The risk of becoming obese increases by a whopping 400 percent!

**Side effects and symptoms of artificial sweeteners:**
* Altered brain chemistry
* ADD, depression, psychiatric and behavioral problems
* Birth defects, cancer
* Abdominal bloating and edema
* Brain seizures and tumors
* Cravings – artificial sweeteners trigger an increase in appetite without satisfying hunger and interfere with your body's ability to feel full, causing one to overeat
* Increased risk of heart disease
* Elevated blood sugar, insulin resistance and diabetes
* Insomnia
* Migraines
* Mimics Parkinson's disease, chronic fatigue, fibromyalgia, M.S., and Alzheimer's disease
* Muscle spasms
* Rashes and hives
* Weight gain – *resulting in obesity*

Do you really love your diet soda that much? For every diet soda you drink per day, you are 65 percent more likely to become overweight during the next seven to eight years, and 41 percent more likely to become obese. Diet soft drinks and artificial sweeteners are a sure-fire way to increase your chances of getting fatter and sicker.

Healthier sweeteners include stevia, xylitol, Lo Han extract, coconut nectar, coconut sugar, raw organic honey, black molasses and real maple syrup.

## Vegetable oils and polyunsaturated fatty acids (PUFAs)

PUFAs, including corn, safflower, sunflower, canola, soy, peanut and cottonseed oils, are *not* the healthy alternatives the media would have you believe them to be.

Vegetables oils, loaded with omega-6 fatty acids, are rancid oils that are treated with deodorizers. The fast food-industry uses and reuses these toxic oils to fry french fries and other deep-fried food items. The majority of processed and packaged foods contain vegetable oils. Egg substitutes, also known as plastic eggs, are made with toxic vegetable oils. For a healthier option, eat the real thing – organic, pastured eggs. Pastured eggs are chicken eggs that have been harvested from chickens allowed to roam in open pasture as opposed to being kept in confinement and fed primarily grains.

While a very small amount of omega-6 fats are necessary for health, excessive intake, as in the average American diet, has been shown to promote inflammation and increase appetite and weight. Consuming vegetable oils contributes to an overproduction of endocannabinoids, a substance similar to what is found in cannabis (THC) that signals hunger to the brain, creating the urge to overeat.

Excessive intake of polyunsaturated fats and vegetable oils increase your risk of:
* Cancer
* Heart disease
* Learning disabilities
* Lung damage
* Inflammation
* Digestive disorders
* Immune system dysfunction
* Liver dysfunction
* Elevated uric acid levels
* Weight gain

Avoid all products with corn, canola and soybean oil and other PUFAs. The end result of consuming these toxic oils is extensive oxidative damage to your cells. Switch to simple, wholesome butter, coconut oil, olive oil and other truly healthy fats for a Hot 'n Healthy Body (see *Chapter 13*).

## Frankenfats

Partially hydrogenated oils and trans-fatty acids (TFAs), also known as frankenfats, are oils that have been chemically altered in order to make them stable at room temperature. You'll find partially hydrogenated oil in thousands of food items, such as chips, breakfast cereals, cookies, crackers and hundreds of other processed foods.

TFAs are proven to cause heart disease and diabetes, increase body fat suppress thyroid function and accelerate aging. Restaurant food, especially from fast-food chains, often serve food loaded with trans-fats. Just a few consequences of a diet high in trans-fats include:

* Arthritis
* Cancer
* Decreased immune function
* Decreased IQ – learning disabilities
* Elevated blood pressure and heart disease
* Free radical production
* Impaired neurological and visual development of fetus
* Increased inflammation
* Liver damage
* Lower testosterone
* Obesity
* Osteoporosis
* Type 2 diabetes

## Processed soy

When it comes to soy, much of what we read and hear about comes from those who market it. Before you mix up a soy protein shake, snack on a soy protein bar or pour yourself a glass of soy milk, consider this – unfermented, processed soy is deficient in amino acids, is estrogenic, disrupts sex hormones, is toxic to infants, shrinks the brain, contains high levels of aluminum and inhibits the thyroid. Drinking just two glass of soy milk daily for one month alters a woman's menstrual cycle and lowers testosterone in men.

Soybeans also contain lectins, compounds that bind with intestinal cells and interfere with nutrient absorption and other compounds such as saponins, lipoxidase, phytoestrogens and goitrogens, whose anti-nutritional effects are not known. It is especially important that those who are experiencing thyroid dysfunction completely avoid soy as it binds thyroid hormones and thyroid medication, rendering them ineffective. Soy also blocks the uptake of minerals, especially iodine, which is necessary for healthy thyroid function.

Before we jump off the soy bandwagon altogether, there are a few redeeming qualities to soy, found primarily in organic and fermented, non-GMO soy products like tempeh, miso, natto and soybean sprouts. If you want to reap some of the health benefits from soy, stick to these four forms. The fermentation process neutralizes the naturally occurring high level of toxins (phytic acid and other digestive inhibitors) found in soy, but not the phytoestrogens.

In the interest of overall health and fat loss, it is best steer clear of any product containing soybean oil and soy protein. In addition, avoid soy milk, tofu and other unfermented, soy-based ingredients – often disguised as health foods – such as soy veggie burgers, soy ice cream and soy cheese. These and many other processed soy products are made from genetically modified soybeans and subjected to hexane, a chemical solvent, and other artificial food ingredients used to enhance their taste.

> *Unfermented, genetically-modified and processed soy is unhealthy for anyone at any age!*

## Sodium chloride

Commonly known as commercial table salt, sodium chloride is highly processed and contains chemicals, additives and aluminum, which are toxic and cause neurodegenerative disorders. Opt for a healthier version such as Bragg's amino acids, Himalayan salt or unprocessed Celtic sea salt.

## Genetically modified organisms (GMOs)

A GMO is a plant, animal or microorganism whose genetic code has been altered, subtracted or added (either from the same species or a different species) in order to give it characteristics that it does not have naturally.

Genetic engineering (GE) or genetic modification (GM) of food involves the laboratory process of artificially inserting genes into the DNA of food crops or animals. They are produced to meet a particular need, such as making the grain cheaper or more resistant to insects.

GE foods appear to your body as foreign invaders rather than food, triggering an immune attack that can lead to chronic inflammation, severe infertility problems and may even cause the bacteria in your body to produce and release a pesticide in your own stomach. Europe requires labeling of all genetically modified food items; however, the U.S. does not.

Ninety percent or more of all corn, soy, sugar beets, cottonseed and canola grown in the United States is genetically modified. These items should be avoided at all costs.

## Monosodium glutamate (MSG)

MSG is a chemical food additive and an excitatory neurotoxin, excitotoxin. An excitotoxin is a chemical that penetrates certain brain regions and causes a brain cell to become overexcited, fire uncontrollably and rapidly destroy neurons, leading to cell damage and death. MSG has been linked to weight gain, seizures, rashes and hives, depression, panic attacks, migraines, hormone damage, neurodegenerative conditions and other serious disorders.

MSG is used in many processed foods as a taste enhancer and has over 50 different names, such as hydrolyzed and autolyzed proteins and yeast extract, that are used to disguise it on food labels. Avoid anything labeled autolyzed or hydrolyzed.

## Dyes and food colorings

Blue 1, 2; Red 3, 40; Green 3 and Yellow 5, 6 and others are derived from petroleum. Many of these dyes and colorings are contaminated with aluminum. There is evidence that food coloring and food additives contribute to behavioral problems in children, depression, hormonal dysfunction, migraines and even cancer.

Take home message: Stay away from any product listing an ingredient with a color plus a number.

## Label awareness

Keep in mind that just because a food item is labeled organic, sugar-free, gluten-free, dairy-free or fat-free does not mean it's healthy. Such a label should not be perceived as the "green light" to an all-you-can-eat food item. For many products, it's simply deceptive marketing. Some foods you think are healthy for you contain more sugar than a candy bar. For example, a fat-free cookie is sugar and refined grains with zero nutritional value. On the other hand, an avocado is full of fat and nutrients, and much healthier than a fat-free, chemical-laden energy bar.

## Revolution Solutions

Choose to shop at your local farmers' markets, natural health food stores, Mother's Markets, Trader Joe's, Whole Foods and local food cooperatives for the best selection of natural, healthy foods. Stick to nutrient-rich real food, which is usually found on the outer perimeter aisles of the supermarket.

Become an avid and dedicated label reader! If you buy any items in a box or package, always read the list of ingredients on every product.

Wheat, sugar, corn syrup and HFCS, hydrolyzed yeast (MSG), vegetable oils, aspartame, sucralose and partially–hydrogenated oils are just a few things an informed label reader will look for and avoid like the plague.

Completely remove these appetite stimulants from your diet: wheat, gluten, processed foods, vegetable oils, artificial sweeteners and all flour-based foods. Focus on eating wholesome, nutrient–rich, fresh foods. This is the best way to avoid toxic, harmful ingredients.

# Chapter 8

## DETOXIFICATION FOR A HOT 'N HEALTHY BODY

E very day we're exposed to various toxins and chemicals as a result of the food we eat, the air we breathe, alcohol, prescription and OTC drugs, the environment, products we use on our skin and so much more. We're exposed to over ten pounds of toxic food additives every year! Over time, these toxins accumulate in our bodies, often hidden, and can manifest themselves symptomatically as insomnia, fatigue, digestive problems, liver congestion, hives, aches and pains, chronic disease, excess body fat and even cancer.

We're literally swimming in a sea of chemicals that adversely affect our health, energy levels and metabolism, creating great stress on our bodies and weakening our immune systems. Toxic overload primarily targets the liver, brain and adipose tissue, collectively making it difficult to lose body fat. When your body's natural detoxification pathways (liver, kidneys, skin and intestinal tract) become overloaded with an accumulation of toxins, they can trick the body into thinking it is under attack and trigger an increased autoimmune response. In addition, the chemical signals between cells become blocked and produce hormone imbalances.

Toxins accumulate in the body's fat tissue and ultimately lead to weight loss resistance. In overweight individuals, stubborn fat may not want to budge as the cells desperately hold onto fat in an attempt to protect the body from the stress and adverse reactions that may occur from the release of these stored toxins.

## Heavy metal body burdens

Heavy metals are a major source of toxic overload that often go undetected. Many research studies in the U.S. and Europe have linked heavy metal toxicity with a wide range of illnesses and health conditions, including neurological degeneration, Alzheimer's disease, Parkinson's disease, thyroid disorders, obesity, autoimmune diseases, Candida, autism, ADD, joint problems and cancer. Symptoms are often silent and ultimately detrimental to health.

*I highly encourage all of my clients to test for and rule out heavy metal body burdens.*

**Potential sources of toxic heavy metals:**

* Mercury amalgams
* Refined chocolate
* Fish (especially tuna)
* Exhaust and pollution
* Prescription drugs
* Fertilizers and pesticides
* Housecleaning products

* Cosmetics, hair dyes
* Infant formulas
* Paint
* Tattoos
* Processed wheat
* Unfiltered water
* Some protein powders

The liver performs over 500 known functions, including hormone regulation, detoxification, metabolism and bile production. It also filters, regulates and stores blood. The liver is involved with digestion, the hormone system, blood sugar control, and protein and fat metabolism.

All toxins brought into the body have to be processed by the liver. A consequence of a congested liver is excess weight through fluid retention, cellulite and bloating as the body attempts to protect itself by neutralizing the negative effects of the toxic overload. The liver converts harmful chemicals into water-soluble molecules that are released during elimination (one of the reasons why it is so important to have daily bowel movements). When the liver weakens in its ability to detoxify these chemicals, they overflow into the body.

Toxic overload leads to weight loss resistance, organ and gland dysfunction, premature cell death and an increased risk of disease.

According to Mitchell Ghen, D.O., Ph.D., president of the Anti-Aging Academy and pioneer of stem cell research, "*If you breathe, you need to detox*"! Detoxing is simply a term that implies reducing the toxic load from the body's natural system and functions through lifestyle adjustments and diet modifications.

When you detox, toxins are eliminated from the liver first via the bile. Detoxing gives your body a chance to rest, clear out toxins and become nourished. Detoxification is essential for hormonal regulation, deep sleep, optimal digestion and fat loss. Another positive result is that detoxification can clear and refresh our minds. The process of detoxification occurs by first removing and eliminating toxins, followed by nourishing and providing the body with healthy nutrients.

By supporting a healthy liver and a healthy gut, another major organ of detoxification and elimination, toxins move through and out of the body, minimizing toxic overload and excessive DNA damage. A healthy liver is also critical in detoxifying human estrogens and xenoestrogens.

The detoxification process is unique to each individual due to differences in biochemical makeup, level of toxic build-up, stress levels and medical history. Detoxification reactions can occur when the body is releasing toxins. This is called a healing crisis. Another common cause of the healing crisis has to do with the dying off of certain pathogenic organisms in the body. These organisms can be Candida yeast infections, viruses and bacteria.

The symptoms of detoxing experienced during the healing crisis are highly variable to each individual. Some individuals may experience headaches, fatigue, skin breakouts or body aches. These symptoms are primarily the effects of the detoxification in the healing process and should be considered natural and healthy – a sign of progress and an indication that you're on the right path to optimal health!

## Detox solutions for a Hot 'n Healthy Body at any age

There are numerous solutions for healthy detoxification – many of which can also be adopted as part of a healthier lifestyle. You will reduce your toxic load; experience better sleep, increased energy and alleviation from constipation, bloating and puffiness; balance hormones and lower body fat with the following simple lifestyle adjustments and diet modifications:

*   Consume an appropriate amount of clean, filtered water every day. Your body is 85 percent water. Physiologically, water works as a catalyst to the majority of bodily functions. Water consumption is especially important for eliminating toxins, easing stress placed upon the liver and kidneys, losing body fat, and more importantly, keeping fat off.

*   Add the juice from a fresh lemon or lime to your water, especially before meals. This alkalizes your system, supports digestion, promotes bile production and stimulates liver enzymes, increasing the body's ability to cleanse itself of toxins.

*   Use organic, raw and unfiltered apple cider vinegar, which is rich in enzymes and enhances detoxification and cleansing of the kidneys and liver. Apple cider vinegar mixed with olive oil and herbs is a healthy dressing for salads or veggies. Also, try mixing two teaspoons of apple cider vinegar with six ounces of water and sip before meals.

*   Avoid low-calorie diets while detoxing. Diets are a major stressor to your body, damaging your metabolism, creating hormonal disruption, causing muscle loss, increasing fat storage, and consequently adding extra pounds once you stop the diet.

*   Keep a food journal. Research shows that people who journal what they eat lose twice as many pounds *and* make healthier food choices. This is especially helpful during your detox.

* Reduce your intake of alcohol. Excessive alcohol consumption not only disrupts your blood sugar and your hormones, it causes dehydration, toxic overload and free radical damage to your liver; stimulates appetite; and adds inches to your waistline.

* Drink more tea, specifically green and white tea. Green tea is loaded with catechins, a type of plant antioxidant that has been shown in studies to eliminate fat accumulated in the liver, prevent liver damage from alcohol, and encourage healthy liver function. Other teas that are especially beneficial for detoxing include pau d' Arco tea and dandelion tea.

* Opt for organic over commercially-raised, non-organic foods. Start with organic, grass-fed beef and bison, free-range poultry and pastured eggs. Adequate protein intake and specific nutrients are required for the detoxification process to transpire.

* Avoid frankenfoods and frankenfats – vegetable oils, processed soy, processed grains, sugar, soda, pasteurized dairy, artificial sweeteners, high fructose corn syrup, table salt, grains, wheat and gluten. These items increase toxic overload in your body and reduce your liver's ability to detoxify.

* Increase consumption of fiber. Include a variety of leafy greens, low-sugar fruits and plenty of red, green and yellow veggies in your diet. Vegetables and leafy greens – watercress, kale, mustard greens, bitter gourd and dandelion – contain chlorophyll and are natural detoxifiers that encourage the removal of toxins, cleanse the liver and help keep your liver functioning properly. Drinking freshly juiced vegetables or green smoothies further supports the detoxification process, and as a bonus you'll reap additional benefits of more veggies and fiber in your diet.

* Drink a tablespoon of olive oil with the juice of a fresh lemon to encourage elimination, stimulate bile production and excrete toxins from your liver.

* Many herbs and spices enhance detoxification – garlic, ginger, cilantro, turmeric, cayenne, parsley, dandelion and aloe vera.

* Eat three smaller meals instead of fasting for days on end. Always eat a breakfast that includes an organic protein source. The amino acids found in protein stimulate the detoxification process. A protein-deficient diet inhibits the detoxification of environmental toxins and pollutants.

* Refrain from eating after 8:00 p.m. Your body wants to rest and detox later in the evening, not digest food. Eating too close to bedtime minimizes the detoxification process and disrupts sleep.

* Keep a regular sleep schedule. Go to bed and wake up at the same time every day. Ideally, asleep by 10:00 p.m. and awake at 6:00 a.m. During these hours of sleep, your body repairs physically and psychologically balancing hormones, regenerating and repairing. If you're extremely active, more sleep may be needed.

* Minimize exposure to electromagnetic fields (EMFs), which can trigger serious symptoms, including fatigue, headaches, confusion and memory loss in people who are electrosensitive. Simple solutions to reduce EMF exposure: remove all electrical devices from your sleeping area; avoid use of electric blankets and electric heating pads; avoid setting your laptop computer directly on your lap; avoid carrying your cell phone in your pocket or on your hip; stop using the microwave oven; and switch out fluorescent light bulbs for incandescent bulbs. If you live near power lines, consider relocating.

* Surround yourself with like-minded people and form win-win relationships. Determine who is trustworthy and displays character traits of integrity, honesty and authenticity. Consider dissolving any relationship that does not lift you up or serve you in a positive light. Minimize time spent with people, places or things that are low-vibration and negative. Enjoy supportive relationships that nourish your soul and make you feel good.

* Detox your mind. Thoughts are very powerful and can control many aspects of your life, including your health. Over time, emotional stress and negative thoughts can create toxicity. To be healthy, harmony must exist in thought, feeling and physical action. Detoxifying the mind challenges us to dissolve away self-limiting and self-sabotaging beliefs. Keep your conscious mind filled with creative, positive, peaceful and productive thoughts.

* Practice positive affirmations daily. Express gratitude every day. Write five things you are grateful for daily in your gratitude journal. This simple task encourages natural production of serotonin.

* Pamper your skin. Your skin is a major organ of detoxification. It is estimated the skin has the capacity to eliminate over one pound of waste per day. Saunas, especially infrared saunas, accelerate the release of toxins.

* Dry skin brushing before a shower stimulates the lymphatic, immune and nervous systems; enhances proper organ function; helps reduce cellulite; improves circulation; and promotes a greater release of toxins. Starting at your feet, brush in upward strokes toward the heart. A dry skin brush is a hygienic tool specifically designed and used to exfoliate the skin.

* Practice deep, full diaphragmatic belly breathing a minimum of two to five minutes daily. Deep breathing is highly beneficial for the removal of toxins as well as increasing energy, improving mood, calming the mind, shifting the autonomic nervous system and enhancing appearance.

* Get your sweat on with your favorite workout. Exercise is a natural form of detoxification. Any type of movement, from brisk walking to high intensity intervals or strength training, is highly beneficial to cleanse the body of toxins.

* Practice yoga, Qi gong or bounce on a rebounder. Rebounding on a mini trampoline is extremely beneficial for every cell and organ in your body. Doing so stimulates the lymphatic system, increases circulation and boosts the immune system.

* Dispose of toxic household products. Switch to natural cleaning products such as white vinegar and baking soda. Use organic skin care products that are void of chemicals. Swap out plastic storage containers and plastic water bottles for ceramic, glass, or other eco-friendly materials. Replace Teflon cookware with stainless steel or a brand that is free of heavy metals or harmful chemicals.

* Try fasting overnight. Overnight fasting means your last meal of the day is at 6:00 p.m. You forego any late-night snacks after dinner and resume eating at breakfast the next morning. Overnight fasting boosts your metabolism and allows your body to shift into a fat burning zone without dieting.

* Reward yourself. Take time to rest without feeling guilty. Get your daily dose of sunshine (vitamin D). Indulge in a warm bath with Epsom salts, baking soda and a relaxing essential oil such as lavender. Schedule a massage or spend time in a sauna, which increases the effectiveness of detoxification by releasing toxins from your body. Pay attention by listening to your gut (intuition), and give your body, mind and soul the love and support it needs.

## Detox supplements for a Hot 'n Healthy Body at any age

A tailored supplement regime will enhance the detoxification process:

* Alpha lipoic acid (R-ALA), a powerful antioxidant
* L-carnitine, helps detox heavy metals from the brain
* Essential fatty acids
* Fiber powders (soluble fiber)
* Green drinks
* HCL – Digestzymes
* Magnesium
* Milk thistle extract (silymarin)
* N-acetyl-cysteine (NAC), an amino acid with antioxidant and liver-protecting effects
* Probiotics
* Vitamin B6 phosphate
* Vitamin D

Your liver requires magnesium and B vitamins, particularly B6, to detoxify estrogens and cortisol.

You can take it a step further with a 10-day detox program developed by Abbas Qutab, M.D. This healthy program is valuable to all individuals, including busy people, because they are able to conduct life normally while following the program. Many individuals suffering from allergies, sinusitis, fatigue and other chronic complaints have experienced gratifying results with the 10 Day Detox Program.

Prior to starting any detox program, consult with your healthcare provider.

# CHAPTER 9

## FAT LOSS RULES, THOUGHTS AND VALUES FOR A HOT 'N HEALTHY BODY

Whether your goal is to lose five percent body fat, fit into a size 8 jean or adopt healthier eating habits overall, a crucial element is love and acceptance of yourself as you are right now. Learning to relate to yourself in a more loving and gentle manner will encourage a healthier body image – an important aspect of maintaining fat loss.

Whenever you have an emotion, there is a thought that interprets it. Emotions can be influenced by hormones and neurotransmitters. In psychology, emotion is often defined as a complex state of feeling, resulting in physical and psychological changes that influence thought and behavior. Emotions and lifestyle choices determine the outcome of your weight, well-being and overall health more than anything else.

The body is inseparable from the mind. Unhealthy, negative thoughts may manifest as poor posture, chronic aches and pains, elevated blood pressure, an autoimmune disease or unwanted body fat. When you change your thinking process, you can alter your brain's neurochemistry and ultimately your physique.

The relationship between food and eating often reveals a deeper awareness and understanding of what is happening subconsciously. The quality and types of food you eat have a direct influence on your thoughts, emotions and energy.

Scientist and author Candace Pert says, "If you truly want to understand what's happening in your subconscious, look at your physical body. The physical body is where unresolved emotions and mental patterns accumulate." When you release thoughts and emotions that no longer serve you, transformation begins to happen.

A study published in *Psychological Science* found that women who wrote about their most important values, such as close relationships, music or spirituality, lost more weight than women who did not process their values through writing. In addition, numerous studies have found that simply thinking briefly about your values can have a profound effect on situations.

The greater the outer change or physical change you wish to manifest, the inner change or emotional change must be even greater. Serious intention and desire for personal growth and change to evolve requires emotional motivation.

> When you start to "BE" that thought and "DO" that specific action, you will "HAVE" inevitable transformation.

Your decision to change starts with a thought. Therein, behavioral change takes place. Mentally prepare yourself to get healthy. Start by focusing on your intention. An intention is a subtle energy that attracts what you want. It is a decision within that transforms your goal into reality.

You are more likely to change your behavior when you focus on your intention and actually write your goals down. Be very clear, specific and detailed when writing your goals and vision. Identify any obstacles or destructive thought patterns to obtaining your goals. Visualize yourself following through with your goals so success is not only possible, it's inevitable. For example, you might decide in advance that every time you're tempted to eat ice cream after dinner, you will take a twenty minute walk or soak in a hot bath instead. When this craving arises, it's a signal for you to take a walk or soak in a warm bath rather than eat the ice cream.

My experience for successfully transforming any area in life, and also the focus in my first book, *The Power of 4,* is to implement two healthy changes every week. Each day of the week you focus on keeping your commitment to these two specific goals. Small, incremental changes ultimately result in life-altering rewards that are absolutely profound and definitely worth every bit of your effort. I encourage you to share and communicate your goals and plan of action with friends, co-workers and family. Doing so reinforces your commitment to attain your goals.

Remember that growth is incremental. Even the longest journey begins with one small step. Always plan to succeed. Break free of old patterns and limiting beliefs. Believe in yourself to achieve results.

> *Focus on the positive reward of a behavior rather than the sacrifice or effort.* ♥

## Eat What You Love – Love What You Eat

### The 90/10 *Revolution Solution*

Dieting and avoiding your favorite foods and treats may lead to weight loss initially, but in reality this will not work long-term. Remember, your goal is long-term, permanent fat loss – a lifestyle, not a diet. When you align yourself and put forth the effort to follow the principles in the *Fat Loss Revolution* 90 percent of the time, consider yourself successful on your fat loss journey.

The *Fat Loss Revolution* is a process geared toward genuine health and authentic vitality with a bonus of losing body fat.

Rigid restrictions and the all-or-nothing approach do nothing more than set you up for failure. As you progress on your fat loss journey, let go of the need to be perfect 100 percent of the time. Rather, focus on making healthier choices 90 percent of the time. The remaining 10 percent of the time allow for those occasions when you wish to sensibly enjoy a glass of wine or three to four bites of your favorite dessert or a holiday treat.

Be aware that if you delve into the 10 percent zone and indulge in a specific food that your body does not handle well, such as sugars and chemically-processed carbohydrates, you will probably feel the negative effects from ingesting these foods and may experience less than desirable symptoms. This is just another confirmation of the toxic effects certain foods have on your body and biochemistry.

Personally, I am not a proponent of "everything in moderation," especially for those who have diabetes or metabolic syndrome, or those who claim to have tried everything to lose fat and nothing has worked. These individuals likely have a damaged metabolism, are weight loss resistant *and* insulin resistant.

Moderation drives these individuals into a "crave fest" when sugar is eaten. A vicious cycle takes place in which they crave sugar, end up eating more sugar, crash, crave more sugar…and the pattern continues. For them, the insulin roller coaster is set into motion, sabotaging every bit of their fat loss efforts. If you find yourself in this category, limiting sugar and processed carbohydrates is crucial to re-programming and balancing your hormones in order to fuel the fire in the fat burning furnace.

Ask yourself: Is the short-term satisfaction from the sugar-laden food worth it? Make a decision to fuel and nourish your body to feel good. Re-focus your energy right back into your 90 percent zone.

* Pay attention to what you eat and portion sizes.
* Focus on nutrient-dense, wholesome foods.
* Continue to log your meals in your food journal.
* Make a habit to read the list of ingredients, often found in super-small print, on every item.
* If you plan to eat one of your favorite treats, do so without guilt or torturing yourself, but *stop* after three or four bites.
* Be prepared and have snacks that are high in fiber and protein readily available, which will stabilize blood sugar.
* Remove trigger foods from your home.
* Avoid buying foods that you know will cause you to binge uncontrollably.
* Remove the jar of candy from your desk or work area.

Anything is doable if you are committed to doing it and believe in yourself. I promise that you will look and feel so much better; your skin will look vibrant and more youthful; bloating, aches, pain, and excess belly fat often disappear; and as a bonus result you'll lose even more body fat!

## Healthier *Revolution Solution* alternatives

| *Eat this –* | *Instead of this –* |
|---|---|
| Eggs, nitrate-free turkey or chicken sausage, blueberries and walnuts | Cereal, donuts or bagel |
| Seltzer water with flavored stevia | Soda |
| 70 percent dark chocolate square with a handful of almonds | Candy bar |
| Chicken, avocado and pecans wrapped in a collard green leaf | Sandwich with luncheon meat and mayonnaise |
| Kale chips or celery with almond butter | Potato chips |
| Guacamole and red bell peppers | Chips and salsa |
| Almond or coconut milk | Cow's milk |
| Spaghetti squash | Pasta |
| Extra-virgin olive oil and fresh-squeezed lemon | Bottled salad dressings |
| Almond butter | Peanut butter |
| Organic butter | Margarine or butter sprays |
| Free-range, organic, pastured eggs | Frankeneggs (egg substitues) |
| Coconut flour, almond or flax meal | Flour, including wheat flour |
| Protein shake with cocoa, stevia and almond or coconut milk | Chocolate milk shake |
| Quinoa flakes | Quick oats |
| Dark leafy greens | Iceberg lettuce |

# Faster Fat Loss – Be Present in Mind, Body and Soul

*Mindfulness is an "awareness of present experience, with acceptance." Christopher Germer, PhD.*

Many people operate on autopilot throughout the day, and especially during mealtime. Due to the fast-paced, on-the-go schedules they attempt to maintain, many of them end up multi-tasking while they eat.

Your brain and stomach communicate feelings of fullness after approximately 20 minutes. During this time, receptors inform the brain that your body is receiving nutrients by sending hormone signals. Eating on the run, in your car, while watching television or as you check your emails or iPhone result in mindless eating. Studies show over 40 percent more food is eaten while watching television. These distractions trigger you to unconsciously eat more and more food with no attention to portion size. This happens because certain hormones have not had sufficient time to send the correct message.

**Prioritize mealtime.** Resolve to set aside a specific time to eat where you can sit down and dine in a relaxing environment with a calm state of mind. This will make your dining experience more pleasurable. Take a moment and silently express gratitude for the meal you are about to consume.

Plan 20 minutes to sit down and enjoy your meal. Slow down and enjoy your food. When you eat slower, your brain is fooled into thinking that you've eaten more. Set your utensil down after three or four bites of food. Savor each and every bite. Breathe. Breathe again.

Be fully present, conscious and mindful while eating. With conscious control, you become aware of the actual experience of eating. You will notice the food on your plate, savor each bite and essentially taste the flavor and experience the texture of the food. As a consequence, you will consume less food because your brain registers a signal that you are full and satisfied.

The digestive process is 30 to 40 percent less effective when your mind is tuned out during mealtime. To encourage healthy digestion, it is ideal to eat your meals in a pleasant, peaceful environment rather than a hectic one. This means turning off the television, computer, your cell phone and other distractions that trigger mindless eating. Avoid reading stressful news, listening to chaotic music or engaging in a stressful conversation while eating.

Digestion begins in the mouth. Chew your food thoroughly (i.e., approximately 20-30 chews for a piece of meat). When your food isn't thoroughly chewed, the nutrients are not absorbed, you become malnourished and eventually end up with digestive ailments. In addition, this practice signals your body to store fat because the nutrients are not broken down properly, inhibiting absorption. Your body then thinks it's deprived and creates a sense of perceived famine. In fact, people who devour their food are two and a half times more likely to suffer from type 2 diabetes than those who take their time, eat slowly and chew their food.

Digestion and assimilation of food improves tremendously when you take the time to chew your food until it's liquefied before swallowing. You will also eat less and absorb more nutrients.

Try this simple exercise: eat a meal with your eyes closed, or better yet, blindfolded. You will be amazed at the amount of food left on your plate because the visual element is eliminated and your brain is actually communicating to your stomach that it's satisfied. Or, try using your non-dominant hand to hold your utensil, or opt for chopsticks. These simple mind tricks may just slow you down enough to not only enjoy your meal, but absorb the nutrients as well.

**Avoid nibbling.** Stop eating before you're full. Get up from the table and to put away any leftovers. This will prevent any temptation to nibble.

**Take a walk** once you've completed your meal to enhance digestion. Reflect on how nutritious the meal was that you just ate.

**Lose more weight with a food journal.** Keep a daily food journal of everything you eat and drink. Individuals who journal what they eat *lose twice as much weight* and make much healthier food choices than those who do not keep a journal. This simple task will help identify any trigger foods, and is especially helpful for ruling out intolerant foods.

Journaling is an effective way to get in touch with your emotions, feelings and relationship with food.

Start tracking your food intake on a piece of paper you carry in your purse or pocket, in a spiral notebook, on a mobile app, or in a Word document or an online program. Be honest, accurate and consistent. Record every morsel that goes into your mouth, including beverages. Also, document the amount and any other details you wish to track. Doing so is an extremely valuable exercise that creates a system of awareness and accountability. The feedback will be a very beneficial exercise to help identify and change unhealthy behavior patterns of poor food choices, eating too much and eating mindlessly in connection with negative feelings and emotions.

> *Be fully present in mind, body and soul*
> *during mealtime.*

## Mealtime Solutions

### The *Fat Loss Revolution* plate using the PVFC method

The PVFC Method is an acronym for a simple technique to help you remember how to prioritize your food options when planning your meals and what should be on your plate.

| PVFC stands for – | |
|---|---|
| P | Protein |
| V | Vegetable |
| F | Fiber and Fat |
| C | Carbohydrate |

Start with "P." Your first priority is to focus on a source of protein to include at your meal. Half of your plate will be a quality source of protein.

Follow with "V." Determine a vegetable: either a non-starchy vegetable or a dark, leafy green. This also falls under the "F" category as a fiber source.

In addition to fiber, "F" also includes a healthy source of fat, which could be in a piece of salmon, a slice of avocado or an olive oil-based salad dressing.

Last, is "C," which represents a fibrous, low-glycemic carbohydrate or fruit. To optimize fat loss, limit intake or completely skip the "C" option. Once your fat loss goal has been achieved, limit your intake of carbohydrates to the last meal of the day.

Following the PVFC Method makes it easier to prioritize food choices.

## Healthier mealtime choices

Mealtime while dining out at restaurants can be an obstacle and impede your fat loss efforts simply because you have less control over portion sizes, ingredients used and how the food has been prepared. A study in the *Journal of the Academy of Nutrition and Dietetics* found that individuals who prepared their meals at home lost more weight than those who ate out just once per week. However, when you familiarize yourself with the following tips, occasional meals away from home can be healthy, nutritious and comply with your fat loss lifestyle, keeping you in the zone

A great option is to use some of the available phone apps or websites to search for restaurants that serve healthier options. When browsing a restaurant menu, stick with entrees that are the least processed. Always remember the PVFC Method. Choose items listed as grilled, baked, broiled, fresh, sautéed, blackened, roasted or steamed. Avoid items listed as fried, creamy, battered or breaded.

If the menu option you select includes french fries or coleslaw, ask the server to omit those. Choose to double up on the vegetables instead or opt for a dark, leafy green salad. Inquire whether the restaurant offers wild fish, chicken, grass-fed beef or bison. Ask the server how and with what a dish is prepared.

As a replacement to bottled salad dressings or creamy salad toppings, opt for olive oil with lemon or apple cider vinegar. Fat is required to absorb the nutrients from your salad. Avoid non-fat and low-fat salad dressings that often contain sugar, artificial sweeteners, vegetable oils and other less than desirable ingredients that wreak havoc on your hormones and your waistline.

Remind the server not to bring the bread basket, or if the server brings the bread basket, ask them politely to remove it. Be mindful of portion sizes and avoid overeating. Consider sharing an entrée with a friend, or if the entrée you ordered is too large, ask for a to-go box and package half of your entrée before digging in.

Before dinner, whether at home or at a restaurant, sip on a cup or two of warm water with juice of entire lemon or lime. In a study, those who drank two cups of water before each meal lost an average of five pounds more weight on a 12-week calorie-controlled diet than those who followed the same diet but did not drink the water.

When dining at home, or before you leave home for a restaurant, drink one to three teaspoons of apple cider vinegar mixed in a small amount of water 15 minutes before meals. (This is not recommended for those with ulcers.) Simply doing this lowers the glycemic load of a meal, improves insulin sensitivity and prevents fluctuations in blood sugar that can influence weight loss. The small amount of apple cider vinegar in water taken before meals also supports digestion and absorption of the vitamins and minerals from food, improves satiety and prevents overeating by suppressing appetite.

Avoid drinking sugary beverages altogether. A study in the journal *Advances in Nutrition* reports that consuming sugary beverages such as orange juice with your meal reduces fat oxidation (burning). Instead, drink water or green tea; however, minimize consumption of liquids during mealtime to optimize digestion.

Drinking green tea helps boost your metabolism. The catechins found in green tea have antioxidant, anti-inflammatory, anti-cancer and fat oxidation benefits. Brew your own green tea, or drink freshly brewed green tea. Be sure the tea is organic since numerous brands of tea are laced with toxic pesticides. If you prefer sweetened tea, use Stevia Plus. These green packets or liquid drops are the perfect sweetener option and easy to carry in your purse or wallet.

**Use a smaller plate and a taller glass.** The bigger your dinnerware, the bigger your portion sizes. The same goes for your beverage. Those who drink their beverages from a shorter, fatter glass versus a taller, thinner glass tend to consume more. In the last 50 years, plate size has increased from an average of 9 to 12 inches, while at the same time our waistlines have grown by 6 inches.

A 12-inch plate has 77 percent more surface area than a 9-inch plate and holds about twice as much food. When you use a larger plate, you could potentially end up eating nine to 31 percent more than you typically would using a smaller plate by simply switching from a 12 inch to a 9 inch plate, you will unconsciously consume 20 percent less food. Also, the color of your plate can subconsciously impact food intake. According to a study in the journal, *Appetite*, you'll consume less food when you place your food on a red plate versus a white or blue plate.

**Eat your meal in this order.** Refer to and review the PVFC method. To optimize hormonal balance, produce satiety and increase fat loss as you begin to eat, always eat half of your protein source first, followed by a fibrous vegetable and/or salad, and lastly, an optional carbohydrate such as a sweet potato or yam.

Completely forgo the starchy carbohydrates and stick with protein and fiber from vegetables and leafy greens if you're on a serious fat loss mission. A study in the *Archives of Internal Medicine* found that participants consumed 50 percent more calories when they ate a high carbohydrate food first versus protein. Protein controls the appetite centers of the brain.

Start and end your meal with an intention of gratitude.

**Meal timing and frequency.** A study in the *Clinical Journal of Nutrition* looked at the effects of meal frequency and the relationship to fat burning and insulin sensitivity. The study found increased thermogenesis in those who ate small, regular, frequent meals as compared to those who skipped meals. When meals are skipped, metabolism slows down to conserve energy and fat burning comes to a halt. Additionally, those who have irregular eating patterns tend to have higher cholesterol levels and elevated insulin.

**Include a source of protein at breakfast, lunch and dinner.** Doing so will have a dramatic effect on your metabolism and mood, and a positive influence on fat loss. See *Chapter 3* for more on metabolism.

**Traveling.** Maintaining healthy eating habits during travel can be challenging. To prevent any drawbacks you may encounter, strategic planning can make healthy eating while traveling much easier so you stay on track.

For a lengthy road trip, pack a cooler with healthy snacks that you have prepared ahead of time. Pack your Vitamix or a mini high-powered blender to easily blend a smoothie or protein shake.

If you're flying, pack some healthy snacks that travel well such as nuts or seeds, apples, protein powder, pre-cut veggies, sliced chicken breast, jerky or avocado. Drink plenty of water to remain hydrated.

Check ahead of time with your hotel to see if the room offers a kitchenette, or at least refrigerator.

**Food prep.** How your food is prepared and cooked is an important component to consider for optimal health and fat loss. Many restaurants use cheap vegetable oils, commonly soy and canola. When dining at a restaurant, ask the server what type of oil the kitchen uses to prepare meals.

Avoiding all vegetable cooking oils, including corn, soy and canola oil, is extremely important. These highly processed oils are rancid and genetically modified. Once heated, they become oxidized (see *Chapter 7*). Replace these toxic oils at home with organic, virgin coconut oil, which remains stable and does not oxidize at higher temperatures.

Virtually all nutrients in food are susceptible to damage and destruction from heat. Microwaving foods causes biochemical alterations in amino acids and lipids, and depletes nutrients. Eating microwaved foods causes lymphatic and thyroid disorders, cancer and leukemia.

Advanced glycation end (AGE) products are a class of chemical byproducts that result from the combination of protein and sugar when food is cooked by excessive heat. AGE products can also be formed by the body when too much refined sugar is eaten and elevated blood sugar levels are maintained for too long a time. Food manufacturers intentionally increase the number of AGE products in food, either by adding sugar or by browning food elements. They are trading on the great taste of browned or caramelized food to sell more units. AGE products are toxic to the body.

When you eat foods that are cooked at high temperatures, cellular oxidation, inflammation and aging accelerate. Instead, turn down the heat and extend the cooking time. Ingesting harshly cooked foods promote systemic inflammation and increases risk of diabetes and other diseases.

Opt for alternative cooking methods. Cook with water. Consider steaming, poaching, braising, sautéing, boiling, stewing, stir-frying or use a slow cooker. These gentler methods create more moisture during the cooking process and prevent the loss of nutrients.

AGEs can be minimized by cooking meats with foods containing antioxidant bioflavonoids such as lemon, vinegar, onions, garlic and peppers. When onion and garlic are exposed to heat, the amount of sulfur-containing compounds and the variety of nutrients actually increase.

Avoid using bottled sauces that tend to be high in fat and sugar, which end up producing more AGEs. Instead, marinate foods in olive oil, cider vinegar, garlic, mustard, lemon or lime juice and dry wines. This reduces the AGEs and carcinogens produced from grilling by 90 percent.

Avoid processed foods that are likely to have sugar or browned food elements.

Drink organic green tea, which may prevent AGEs.

Finally, add more raw and steamed vegetables to your diet, which are naturally low in AGEs and contain compounds such as antioxidants that decrease some of the damage from AGEs. Be sure to wash all fruits and veggies prior to using them.

**Dessert**. After dinner, avoid the temptation to indulge in dessert. There will be times when there is a special event to celebrate. In those circumstances, limit yourself to eat three to four bites of dessert, savoring the taste and texture. After three to four bites, be finished. When attending special celebrations, offer to bring your own healthy dessert.

**Alcohol** consumption, in excess, will sabotage and inhibit your hard work and fat loss efforts toward achieving a hot 'n healthy body.

First, let's define the term "excess" as it relates to alcohol. According to the National Institute on Alcohol Abuse and Alcoholism (NIAAA), excessive drinking for men is five or more drinks during any one drinking session, or more than 14 drinks a week. For women, four drinks or more during a day, or more than seven drinks a week, is considered heavy drinking for women.

A study published in the *American Journal of Clinical Nutrition* found that the metabolism of alcohol decreased fat oxidation. The same study found that drinking even as little as one ounce of vodka will slow your metabolism by as much as 73 percent. Your liver cannot metabolize alcohol and fat at the same time. The liver will get rid of the toxic substance (alcohol) first. As a result, fat loss metabolism comes to an abrupt halt when you consume alcohol in excess.

Alcohol increases abdominal fat, especially in men, and inhibits your body's ability to produce fat-burning hormones. On top of that, drinking alcohol lowers your inhibitions and stimulates your appetite, encouraging excessive eating. You'll be less likely to avoid temptation for unhealthy foods and snacks, and unconsciously end up consuming more food – the perfect combination if your goal is a muffin top, spare tire or gynecomastia (male breast development).

In addition, alcohol is estrogenic, increases cortisol and lowers both growth hormone and testosterone. It also causes toxic overload and free radical damage to your liver, and destruction and death to brain cells. Alcohol is a poison that causes dehydration and interrupts the normal stages of restful sleep for up to 72 hours. A Friday alcohol binge will disrupt your sleep until the following Tuesday.

If you wish to drink alcohol, opt for a glass of sulfite-free, organic red wine and limit your consumption to one or two glasses maximum with meals one or two days per week. Spanish and pinot noir wines are rich in antioxidants. Pinot noir contains the highest concentration of resveratrol. Resveratrol is a powerful antioxidant found in the skin of red grapes that comes with a variety of health-promoting benefits. If you do indulge in one or two alcoholic beverages, reduce the toxic overload and drink extra water, or better yet, coconut water, since it's jam-packed with electrolytes. Skip the fruity, syrupy drink mixes that are high in calories and disrupt blood sugar.

People tend to crave alcohol when they're hypoglycemic. The root cause of alcohol cravings stems from nutrient deficiencies, particularly magnesium and trace minerals, B vitamins, essential fatty acids, neurotransmitter imbalances and amino acid deficiencies, specifically L-glutamine, methionine, 5-hydroxytryptophan (5-HTP) and L-tyrosine.

Moderate and sensible alcohol consumption is associated with a reduced risk of developing cardiovascular disease, improved insulin sensitivity and an abundance of other health benefits. However, in excess, alcohol disrupts hormones, sleep and interferes with fat loss. Remember, your goal is to build muscle and lose body fat, which requires that your body be hydrated, well nourished and rested. If you have excess belly fat to lose, it's best to avoid alcohol. While an occasional drink or two will not affect your body negatively, drinking alcohol will prevent you from achieving a hot 'n healthy body.

## Food Addictions, Cravings and Fat Loss

Brain chemistry and food addictions are very complex issues. Michael Pollan, author of *In Defense of Foods,* says certain foods that have been industrially processed, meaning the food is made in a plant, rather than grown on a plant, are biologically addictive. These include sugar-, fat- and salt-laden foods – basically all processed, refined, packaged and fast foods. Combine this with brain signals that stimulate neurochemical reward centers in the brain, and you have a food addiction or food craving.

**Frankenfoods** are foods that have been engineered, processed, genetically modified or contain genetically modified organisms (GMOs). Frankenfoods represent an alarming 98 percent of the food produced and consumed by Americans. Fast foods are the grand master of frankenfoods.

Frankenfood manufacturers include ingredients that have narcotic properties in their products. These toxic psychoactive chemicals bind to opioid receptors in the nervous system which activate a feeling of never being satisfied and trigger cravings to eat more and more food – similar to a drug. These highly addictive ingredients cause depression, fatigue and numerous health problems, and promote fat storage.

> *Food is a drug!*
>
> *Seldom does anyone binge on broccoli or apples. On the other end of the spectrum, frankenfoods such as cookies, ice cream, potato chips, fast foods, sugary snacks and the like, are highly addictive for many individuals.*

## Reasons for cravings and food additions

David Kessler, M.D., former head of the Food and Drug Administration and author of *The End of Overeating,* describes the science of how food is made into drugs by creating foods loaded with sugar, fat and salt, which leads to neuro-chemical addiction.

Foods high in sugar, carbs and fat stimulate your brain's reward centers, specifically dopamine, just like drugs. In fact, sugar is more addictive than cocaine! The more sugar you eat, the more you crave it because overindulgence of sugar can cause insulin resistance.

Drugs addicts, alcoholics and obese individuals all share one thing in common: a lower number of dopamine receptors. Dopamine, a neurotransmitter, is a brain chemical associated with the reward and pleasure center. And, just as the drug addict needs more of the drug over time to create their high, a food addict requires more and more food to induce those feelings of satisfaction. When the initial feeling of getting high subsides, the addict must consume their drug or food of choice just to feel normal.

Certain foods – the kind served at fast-food and chain restaurants – change brain chemistry, triggering a neurological response that stimulates people to crave more food, even if they're not hungry. Rich, sweet and fatty foods stimulate the brain to release dopamine. In the process, these foods rewire the brain and activate the dopamine pathways just at the thought of eating these foods.

Serotonin is another neurotransmitter, also known as the feel-good neurotransmitter, that contributes to feelings of happiness and well-being. Serotonin regulates mood, appetite, sleep, aging and memory, and is involved in the ability to resist impulses.

Serotonin deficiencies can cause your appetite to change – either to no interest in eating or to intense cravings, mainly for high-carbohydrate, high-sugar content foods. The brain tries to use sweets and carbs to increase serotonin levels.

The majority of serotonin (90 percent) is located in the digestive tract. It is imperative to evaluate your GI and digestive function and determine if there is an underlying issue disrupting serotonin production. People with gut dysfunction, and those with Candida overgrowth of yeast or fungus, often experience carbohydrate and intense sugar cravings (see *Chapter 6*).

Unmanaged stress, adrenal dysfuntion and emotional triggers can also cause cravings for carbohydrates, sugary treats or alcohol. Bouts of stress release a flood of cortisol, which directly influences your appetite and cravings for highly palatable foods. A symptom of adrenal burnout is addiction – specifically to stimulants, particularly sugar and caffeine, and as well as salty foods and alcohol.

Blood sugar fluctuations also create ravenous cravings. A drop in blood sugar (hypoglycemia) reduces blood flow to your brain, which causes an individual to make poor food choices. Stabilizing blood sugar and insulin levels must be prioritized. This can be easily remedied by choosing to eat healthier meals and snacks that contain protein.

Micronutrient deficiencies and an insufficient intake of essential fatty acids have a significant influence on cravings. More than 90 percent of individuals are deficient in at least one, if not more, micronutrients. Symptoms of micronutrient deficiencies are different for each person and may include headaches, insomnia, depression, thyroid dysfunction, skin problems, low energy and many other symptoms.

Many women who experience PMS and perimenopause tend to have intense sugar and carb cravings. Cravings themselves are a sign of hormonal imbalances often in conjunction to specific nutrient deficiencies. We crave what our bodies are deficient in. For example, your body may be suffering from adrenal burnout or have a mineral deficiency when you crave salt. Cheese cravings indicate an omega-3 fatty acid imbalance.

Similarly, if you crave chocolate or experience Charlie horses, you're most likely deficient in magnesium.

Sugar, white bread and pasta cravers often need thyroid support to stimulate liver production of bile salts and chromium to thin the bile.

Last, but most certainly not least, is the relationship between food allergies, sensitivities and intolerances to food addictions and cravings.

A sure sign an individual is suffering from a food intolerance is when they want to eat the same favorite 20 or 30 foods over and over and over, day after day after day (see *Chapter 5*).

*The number one cause of a food craving or food addiction is an unidentified food allergy, food intolerance or food sensitivity.*

### Revolution Solutions to conquer food addictions and stop sugar cravings

Solutions to overcome food addictions, avoid giving in to tempting cravings and increasing energy include managing blood sugar and balancing hormonal fluctuations (PMS and peri-menopause), healing adrenal dysfunction, addressing underlying emotions and stress, correcting and balancing nutritional deficiencies and refocusing your mind and energy.

* Don't skip meals. Long periods without food will increase cravings for sugar. And, grabbing an energy bar is not considered a meal. Nip this in the bud by eating real food at breakfast, lunch and dinner that includes protein to prevent fluctuations in blood sugar. As a result, cravings for foods that tend to pack on the fat are greatly reduced.

* Consume a natural source of organic protein at every meal. A protein-rich meal sends signals that travel between your gut and your brain to generate feelings of satiety.

* Eat a breakfast that includes an ample serving of quality protein and healthy fats, such as the Poliquin™ meat and nut breakfast. An example of the Poliquin breakfast would be a buffalo burger and pine nuts or chicken breast and walnuts.

* Eat wholesome, nutrient-rich foods more often. Remember, food is a drug. The list of foods and menu plan found in *Chapter 13* will correct nutrient deficiencies, stabilize your blood sugar and balance your hormones.

* When blood sugar is low, you will end up craving carbs, sugar or alcohol. It is important to eliminate storing poor quality foods such as sugary treats, chips, cookies and the like in your home to avoid the ease of accessibility and the temptation for these foods.

*   Include more soluble, fiber-rich foods in your diet with a variety of fresh vegetables like broccoli, cauliflower and leafy greens including spinach, kale and chard, all which help prevent cravings and control blood sugar.

*   Add raw, organic nuts, chia and flax seeds, avocados, apples and berries to your diet.

*   Plan ahead and prepare snacks that can easily be kept in your purse, briefcase, at your desk or in your car (see *Chapter 13*).

Try some of these simple crave-busters:

*   Simply taking a teaspoon of coconut oil will reduce your craving for sugar.

*   Also, try mixing one tablespoon of organic cocoa powder with a cup of hot water, and sweeten with a packet of SweetLeaf Stevia.

*   Or, take two tablespoons of apple cider vinegar in a glass of water to help eliminate or reduce a sugar craving.

*   Another option is drinking a mixture containing four ounces of water with one teaspoon of L-glutamine.

*   Glutamine is the most abundant amino acid in the human body. One of the most important characteristics of glutamine is that is plays a critical role in glutathione metabolism. Glutamine is also effective for digestive inflammation, repairing the intestinal lining of the gut, protein re-synthesis, and playing a role in immune function. In a double-blind crossover study, supplementation with L-glutamine decreased the desire to drink alcohol in nine out of ten patients. L-glutamine also has blood sugar-stabilizing effects, which helps to eliminate sugar cravings.

* Other crave-busters include cocoa powder and saffron, which is thought to act similarly to a serotonin reuptake inhibitor, a class of compounds typically used as antidepressants in the treatment of depression and anxiety disorders.

* Balance your hormones, specifically insulin and cortisol.

* Identify deeper emotional triggers and deal with stress positively. (*Refer to Chapter 5 for some stress-less solutions.*)

* Start monitoring your diet more closely and eliminate foods you're sensitive or intolerant to. Specifically, avoid wheat, pasteurized dairy, soy, processed and fast foods, and eliminate foods that trigger cravings such as sugar and artificial sweeteners. Sugar is a toxin that is highly addictive.

* Avoid medications, stimulants and excess alcohol consumption, which not only deplete vital nutrients from your body, but also stimulate your appetite, intensify cravings and encourage excessive eating.

* The amount and quality of sleep you get every night has a direct influence on cravings. Make sure you get seven to nine hours of restful sleep every night. When you don't sleep well or skimp on sleep, your appetite increases, especially for sugar, carbohydrates and junk food.

* When you experience an intense craving, shift your mind and focus your energy on healthier, more pleasurable activities. Call a friend. Go for a walk. Light some candles and take a warm bath. Write in your journal about gratifying moments in your life or things, people and places that you love. Read a favorite novel.

* Investigate and rule out gut pathogens including Candida and parasites, which thrive on sugar. Following the *Fat Loss Revolution* eating plan is the first step to healing and starving these sugar-hungry cells.

* Follow the smart workout programs found in *Chapter 11*. When done consistently, the *Fat Loss Revolution* workouts are therapeutically effective for banishing food cravings.

* Commit to a seven-day sugar fast. Although this can be quite challenging for some, the outcome and benefits are huge.

* Work with a qualified practitioner to determine your specific nutrient deficiencies, which are different for each person.

* Specific nutrients, herbs and spices can alleviate food addictions and prevent cravings. These may include:
  - Essential fatty acids
  - Chromium GTF
  - Alpha lipoic acid (R-ALA)
  - Branched chain amino acids (BCAAs)
  - L-glutamine powder
  - High-potency B vitamins
  - 5-HTP
  - Magnesium
  - Vitamin D
  - L-tyrosine
  - Fiber powders
  - N-acetyl-cysteine (NAC)
  - Gymnema
  - Ginseng
  - Fenugreek
  - Cinnamon, cloves

**Reduce sugar cravings with a *Fat Loss Revolution* Smoothie**

* 1 tsp. L-glutamine powder
* 1 tsp. BCAA powder
* 1 tsp. coconut oil or chia seeds
* 1 packet Stevia Plus
* 2 scoops Vital Whey protein
* 1 cup water
* Ice

Blend together in Vitamix or blender. Enjoy!

Also, try the Chocolate Raspberry Cocoa Smoothie. Refer to *Chapter 15* for the recipe.

# CHAPTER 10

---

## HOW FRIENDS SABOTAGE A HOT 'N HEALTHY BODY

C ould your social life, friends and people you surround yourself with affect your behavior by influencing or sabotaging your fat loss efforts? You bet!

There is a powerful link between an individual's weight, what they eat and drink, how much they exercise, and those in their close circle.

Your choices, whether healthy or not, can be swayed or manipulated by people you choose to surround yourself with. For decades, philosophers and sociologists have suspected that behaviors can be contagious. According to research published in the *New England Journal of Medicine,* if your friends or spouse overeat, there is a 57 percent higher tendency that you will overeat as well.

An important fact to consider is whether a particular friend, colleague or family member supports and encourages your healthy lifestyle. Sometimes even a close friend or a loved one can act unintentionally or intentionally as eating behavior saboteurs. Become aware of how others can influence your decisions and efforts – and set boundaries. Shift your mindset and get into the habit of making your own choices when it comes to eating, drinking and exercise. For example, if a co-worker invites you to happy hour, keep your alcohol intake to a minimum. Enjoy one glass of red wine and then switch to water. If happy hour includes a snack, stick with protein-rich options such as shrimp cocktail or chicken skewers with veggies.

You are the sum total of the five people you spend the most time with. Take a moment and reflect. Is your circle of friends optimistic and encouraging? Do they have a positive influence on you in terms of healthy living and eating habits? If not, perhaps it's time to seek others who are compatible, like-minded and understand the value and importance of living a healthy lifestyle.

Choose to surround yourself with individuals who support you and prioritize health: a nutritionist, a fat loss coach, a formal support group, or your friends and family. Having a coach can identify your specific obstacles and what strategies are best for your success. Attend a health workshop or class or consider one-on-one counseling. Associate with others who value their health and practice a similar lifestyle. Doing so creates a healthy connection with others and a positive impact on accountability.

Research has proven that people who join together when their goal is fat loss are more successful in achieving their fat loss goals and live a healthier lifestyle. They tend to experience more dramatic transformations when they have a strong network of like-minded support.

Plan your life in such a way that you are regularly in contact with those who influence you and your behavior positively. The more time you spend with people who support you and share the same behaviors, values and habits as you do, the more likely you will develop and stick with those same characteristics and habits and become a role model for others.

I encourage you to write down your fat loss goals. Be realistic. Share your goals with your close friends. Notice the impact this small act has toward reinforcing success to achieve your fat loss goals. As Mark Twain advised:

> Keep away from people who try to belittle your ambitions. Small people always do that, but the really great make you feel that you, too, can become great. When you are seeking to bring big plans to fruition, it is important with whom you regularly associate. Hang out with friends who are like-minded and who are also designing purpose-filled lives. Similarly, be that kind of a friend for your friends.

*Fat loss is contagious!*

## CHAPTER 11

## REV IT UP WITH INTELLIGENT EXERCISE FOR A
## HOT 'N HEALTHY BODY

The key to an effective exercise program that produces optimal health and results in accelerated fat loss is an intelligently designed program that focuses on intensity, *not duration*. The traditional approach of "more is better" is completely passé. The rate of return is detrimental to not only long-term health, but also achieving permanent fat loss.

The exercise programs found in the *Fat Loss Revolution* concentrate on intentional results that will:
* Boost your metabolism
* Burn more fat
* Increase lean muscle
* Reduce insulin resistance
* Balance your hormones
* Increase bone mineral density
* Improve your energy, mood and self-esteem
* Diminish belly fat
* Enhance strength
* Guarantee RESULTS!

> *An intelligent exercise program that results in fat loss is one that focuses on intensity, not duration!*

## Intelligent exercise Rx

The best type of exercise that is guaranteed to alter your body composition and change your physique is one that consists of resistance strength training with weights and high-intensity intervals, such as sprint intervals. A 2008 study in the journal of *Medicine & Science in Sports & Exercise* found that body composition changes are affected by the intensity of exercise training, strength training and interval training, with interval training being the most effective for reducing total abdominal and subcutaneous fat and losing abdominal visceral fat.

Another study published in the *Journal of Obesity* reported that 12 weeks of high intensity interval training causes significant reductions in total abdominal, trunk and visceral fat, and considerable increases in aerobic power and fat-free mass (muscle). The *Journal of Obesity* also found that the effect of regular aerobic exercise on body fat is negligible.

**Benefits of the *Fat Loss Revolution* exercise Rx include:**

* Improved
    * athletic performance
    * cardiovascular health
    * insulin sensitivity
* Increased
    * aerobic and anaerobic capacity
    * feel-good endorphins
    * metabolism
    * energy
    * fat burning
    * human growth hormone (HGH)
    * lean muscle mass
* Less time spent with greater results
* Reduced inflammation
* Decreased intra-abdominal fat and total body fat

## Long, slow distance (LSD) exercise

Steady-state aerobic or steady-state cardio – also known as long slow distance (LSD) exercise – such as jogging and running is not the best workout or the smartest choice if

* you're limited on time.
* you want optimize hormone balance.
* you want lean cut abs and legs.
* your goal is fat loss.
* you would rather appear lean versus soft and skinny (skinny-fat).
* you want to increase metabolically-active, lean tissue.
* you want to look younger.
* you want a hot 'n healthy body.

The problem with LSD exercise as the only activity of choice is two-fold: whether the intensity is too high or too low, very little, if any, fat is burned. Fat must be converted through a series of enzymes into a substance your body can use.

LSD activity involves the aerobic energy system (type I muscle fibers) only, and neglects the anaerobic energy system (type IIA and IIB muscle fibers). When the type IIA and IIB muscle fibers are activated, higher amounts of exercise-induced growth hormone is released, creating the perfect environment for burning fat.

LSD exercise can cause an insulin resistant or diabetic person to actually become fatter. The *Fat Loss Revolution* exercise prescription, which includes lifting weights and interval training is the better option for an insulin-resistant individual or a diabetic. LSD exercise produces a more rapid decrease in blood sugar than lifting weights. Lifting weights is also associated with less severe drops in blood sugar hours after exercise.

The number of insulin receptors increases when you lift weights, which helps to improve insulin sensitivity. As a result, extra glucose goes into the muscle tissue instead of the fat cells.

When LSD exercise is performed excessively, too hard or as the only mode of activity, the long-term effects can be counterproductive to overall health and body composition.

**Drawbacks of LSD exercise include:**

* Increased inflammation
* Elevated cortisol production
* Excess belly fat
* Hormonal imbalances – lowered testosterone and growth hormone
* Overuse injuries
* Oxidative stress
* Loss of lean-metabolically active muscle tissue
* Accelerated aging
* Increased risk of heart damage
* Adrenal burnout

*If your goal is to*
  * *decrease your body fat composition,*
  * *spend less time and reap greater results,*
  * *keep inflammation at bay,*
  * *have defined abs and leaner legs, and*
  * *transform your body to a hot 'n healthy body,*
*the exercise prescription guaranteed to achieve these results is an intelligently-designed strength training program coupled with sprint intervals, not LSD exercise.*

## Interval training for a hot 'n healthy body

An interval-based training program is nine times more effective for fat loss than endless hours of LSD exercise. A study in *Medicine & Science in Sports & Exercise* indicates that just one 45-minute high-intensity workout will increase resting metabolic rate (RMR) by 37 percent for up to 14 hours after exercise.

Numerous studies continue to confirm that intervals are more efficient and more time effective for fat loss and hormonal balance than LSD activity performed at a lower intensity.

A 1994 study in the journal *Metabolism* monitored two groups of people to evaluate different exercise programs and the effect on metabolism and body fat. One group did steady-state aerobic training for 20 weeks, and the other group did interval training for 15 weeks. Although the results showed that the aerobic group burned 48 percent more calories than the interval group, *the interval group had nine times greater subcutaneous (fat under the skin) fat loss!*

Another study conducted on women between the ages of 22 and 65 showed that two weeks of interval training increased fat oxidation by 36 percent, and these results did not depend on the fitness level of the women before starting the study.

Muscle tissue is metabolically-active and accelerates fat burning. To increase the thermic effect for fat loss to occur, you must increase your muscle mass. This is achieved by lifting weights and interval training.

*Work Out Smarter to Achieve a Hot 'n Healthy Body! Lifting weights, intervals and sprints produce the best results for fat loss in the shortest amount of time, regardless of your conditioning level.*

## Let's get started

Whenever anyone starts a new fitness program, there may be some level of muscle soreness. This is normal, especially for those who have been sedentary for some time. However, if the soreness prevents you from functioning the next day or two, you may have done too much too soon. When in doubt, do less.

> *Those who have been sedentary or those with injuries or other muscular issues should check with a physician before beginning any type of workout, including the exercise programs found in the* Fat Loss Revolution.

## Fitness equipment

Whether you choose to work out at home or at a local health club or gym, the exercise equipment required for the *Fat Loss Revolution* strength training programs and interval fat-blasting REV workouts include:

* Free weights: dumbbells, barbells and weight plates
* Squat rack or power cage
* Pull-up bar
* Pulley cable crossover system
* Jump rope
* Foam roller
* Medicine ball
* Swiss ball
* Jump stretch bands (to assist with chin-ups and pull-ups)
* Optional: kettlebell

**Workout rules for success**

* Approximately 60-90 minutes before your workout, eat a meal that contains protein or opt for a protein shake.
* Drink a minimum of 30 ounces of clean, filtered water *during* your workout.
* Take your pre-workout supplements.
* Do not neglect a proper warm up.
* Focus on intensity, not duration.
* Make each workout count.
* Lift heavy enough weights to stimulate a hormonal response without compromising form and technique.
* Keep a workout journal to record your reps, sets and load.
* Complete your workout with post-exercise nutrition to optimize recovery and protein re-synthesis.
* Avoid drinking sugary beverages or popular energy drinks while working out. Drinking a caloric beverage like orange juice during moderate intensity exercise inhibits fat oxidation by 25 percent.
* Be consistent. No missed workouts.

When you strive to build muscle, lose body fat and enhance recovery, make every effort to maintain a positive protein balance throughout the day, and especially after your workout.

With the appropriate pre– and post–workout nutrition, protein synthesis and fat loss will be maximized. Approximately 80 percent of fat loss results will be related to the foods you eat or don't eat.

A study published *Medicine & Science in Sports & Exercise* concluded that consuming a minimum of 20 grams of whey protein 30 minutes before resistance training boosts metabolism for up to 24 hours after the workout. Consuming 20 grams of whey protein before exercise and another serving afterward will yield the biggest bang-for-your-buck by increasing both fat burning and muscle building.

## Whey protein for a Hot 'n Healthy Body at any age

Whey is one of the highest-quality sources of proteins because of its ideal and abundant profile of branched chain amino acids (BCAAs), which are used to fuel working muscles, stimulate protein synthesis and produce glutathione, a powerful antioxidant.

Consuming whey protein reduces exercise-induced free radicals and oxidative damage and speeds recovery and adaptation to exercise. According to *Alternative Medical Review*, whey protein is an antioxidant and antibacterial that offers immune-enhancing benefits and aids in exercise performance. Australian research shows that supplementation with whey protein improves blood pressure and vascular function in overweight and obese individuals. Yet another study in the *British Journal of Nutrition* demonstrated that supplementation with whey protein improves fasting lipids and insulin levels.

Despite the number of protein powders on the market, not all of them are equal. Many common brands of commercial protein powders are contaminated with toxic heavy metals such as lead, arsenic, cadmium and mercury. As a matter of fact, according to a *Consumer Reports* evaluation, more than 15 of the leading protein powders on the market today contain these toxic chemicals.

Lower quality protein powders and protein drinks are derived from pasteurized, commercial dairy sources and contain lactose and artificial sweeteners. Other common ingredients found in commercial protein powders to avoid include sucralose, soy, corn syrup, maltodextrin, artificial sweeteners, canola oil and vegetable oils.

Always read the list of ingredients on whey products. The longer the list of ingredients, the higher the likelihood is that the product is processed and contains toxic chemicals, cheap ingredients, fillers and artificial ingredients.

Look for high-quality whey protein powders that are organic and derived only from grass-fed cows with absolutely no hormones, steroids, antibiotics, sugars or artificial sweeteners.

Alternative sources to whey protein include rice, pea, hemp, chia and cranberry protein powders. These vegetarian sources of protein powder should be organic, non-GMO and gluten-free.

## Optimize fat loss with pre- and post-workout nutrition

Pre- and post-workout nutrition are important components that will enhance your workouts, optimize fat loss, encourage faster recovery from intense workouts, decrease inflammation and restore protein synthesis.

Recovery capabilities are different for each person and depend upon various factors, such as:

* Age
* Amount of and type of exercise
* Belief in yourself
* Diet and nutrition
* Hydration
* Level of fitness
* Lifestyle (work/job, relationships, etc.)
* Massage, stretching, foam roller and other modes of recovery that are beneficial for your muscles, tissue and nervous system
* Pre- and post-workout nutrition
* Restful sleep every night, seven to nine hours
* Scheduling active recovery days and relaxation exercises
* Stress management
* Supplementation

**Pre-workout fat loss nutrition**

Consume your pre-workout nutrition 30 minutes before your workout:

* Protein, 30-40 grams
* Branched chain amino acid (BCAA) powder, 5-10 grams
* L-carnitine tartrate, 2 grams
* Vitamin C, 500 mg
* Vitamin E, 400 I.U.
* 1 cup of organic, black coffee (optional)

A 2010 study published in *Medicine & Science in Sports & Exercise* demonstrated that consuming 20 grams of whey protein 30 minutes before resistance training boosts metabolism for as much as 24 hours after the completion of the workout and benefits protein synthesis during exercise recovery.

**Post-workout fat loss nutrition**

Consume your post-workout shake within 20-30 minutes after completion of your workout to maximize muscle synthesis, blunt cortisol and optimize recovery.

Protein shake:

* Protein powder (Vital Whey or Whey Cool or Vegetarian Protein Plus), 30-40 grams
* L-glutamine powder, 5-10 grams
* Branched chain amino acid (BCAA) powder, 5-10 grams
* Greens powder, 1 scoop
* Water or coconut water, 12-16 ounces
* Ice

Supplements:

* Vitamin C, 500 mg.
* CoQ10, 100 mg.
* Magnesium glycinate, 400 mg.
* Taurine, 1 gm.

*Please visit PaulaOwens.com/store.html for the pre- and post-workout supplements.*

## Lift weights for a Hot 'n Healthy Body at any age

The *Fat Loss Revolution* workout solution for altering body composition is strength training, especially at higher intensities.

Muscle is your metabolically-active, fat burning tissue. For every additional pound of muscle on your body, you will burn an additional 50 calories per day, whereas each pound of fat burns a trivial two calories daily. Resting metabolic rate (RMR) remains elevated with strength training for 48-72 hours post-workout. This increase in RMR is referred to as excess post-exercise oxygen consumption (EPOC), often referred to as the "afterburn." EPOC is an increased rate of oxygen after strenuous activity.

A study published in the *Journal of the American College of Nutrition* looked at a group of obese individuals who were assigned to one of two exercise routines. One group did LSD exercise (walking, biking or jogging) four times per week while the second group did resistance training three times per week and no LSD exercise. At the end of the 12 week study, even though both groups lost weight, the difference between fat lost versus muscle was significant. The LSD aerobic group lost 37 pounds total, with ten of those pounds lost being lean, metabolically-active muscle tissue. The resistance training group lost 32 pounds and maintained their lean tissue. Not only that, the at-rest metabolic rate of the LSD aerobic group decreased by 210 calories per day whereas the resistance training group increased their metabolism by 63 calories per day. There are hundreds of similar studies on the benefits of strength training for fat loss.

A prevalent mistake routinely made by women in gyms all over the world is that they do not lift heavy enough weights. They tend to perform a high number of repetitions with the pink two to five dumbbells. Females in their twenties, thirties, forties and up often complain that their legs are either fat or thick. Upon observation, these women tend to spend a vast amount of time doing cardio, aerobic classes and LSD-style exercise.

Never or seldom do these women spend any time lifting heavy weight because they fear they will get big and bulky. It seems the heavier the woman is, the lighter the weights she uses. She is afraid that lifting heavy dumbbells will make her even bigger.

Observe the lean, tight and athletically-toned women. More often than not these women lift heavier weights. When women build muscle, their appearance tends to take on a leaner, fit, athletic look. Proper diet, nutrition, hormonal balance and other lifestyle factors found in the *Fat Loss Revolution* must always be factored in.

Heavy strength training stimulates testosterone and growth hormone. Testosterone and growth hormone are key hormones for supporting and building muscle. Growth hormone, released during exercise and sleep, increases fat metabolism and boosts your immune system. Women will not get big and bulky from lifting weights since women have approximately one-tenth the testosterone of males. Due to sarcopenia (see page 10) that occurs as a result of the aging process, strength training is an effective and natural way to offset the decline in testosterone and growth hormone.

Intramuscular and subcutaneous fat diminish when the body is challenged with adequate overload (heavy weights). Continually using light weights and a high number of repetitions will not achieve this effect. The only time lighter weights and higher repetitions are recommended is during the introductory phase for trainees who do not have experience and need to strengthen their joints and tendons first. This initial phase builds a solid foundation that will create quality motor engrams (instructions stored in the brain that tell the body how to perform a specific movement), prevent injuries and ensure proper exercise technique and quality of movement.

The *Fat Loss Revolution* strength training programs involve the major muscles using multi-joint exercises that will force your body to lose the fat reserves and increase muscle mass.

The more muscle you have, the more effectively you will burn fat – providing you are not feasting on carbohydrates, drinking like a fish, sleep deprived or overly stressed.

The best exercises to achieve a Hot 'n Healthy Body are total body strength training exercises such as Olympic lifts, squats, a variety of lunges, dead lifts, stepups and pushing and pulling movements (pullups, pushups, overhead presses) using sand bags, body weight, dumbbells, suspension training (TRX), kettlebells, sleds, pulleys and barbells. These multi-joint exercises have a high metabolic cost, and when done properly they build muscle and increase fat oxidation.

Ideally, strength training routines should be periodized (planned variation and manipulation of intensity and volume) every four to six weeks for consistent change and continued progression. A periodized exercise program increases strength and encourages neuro-muscular adaptations while minimizing boredom and complacency, and prevents plateaus, overtraining, pattern overload and injuries. The older you are in "training years," the more often you will benefit from a change in program design.

The body tends to acclimate quickly to the imposed demands placed upon it. The number one approach to vary a strength training routine is by manipulating the repetitions and sets. Never spend more than four weeks in one repetition zone. Other variables that influence your exercise program design include the exercise selection, order of the exercises performed, length of the rest interval and the tempo of the exercise. The exercise selection should provide progressive overload, intensity and adequate stimuli to your muscular and nervous systems. The *Fat Loss Revolution* strength training programs deliver just that, plus phenomenal results.

*Strength training is essential to achieve permanent fat loss.*

## Fat Loss *Revolution* Strength Training Programs

### Program design instructions

The *Fat Loss Revolution* strength training programs are made up of three phases – Phase 1, Phase 2 and Phase 3. Each phase consists of two workouts, Workout A and Workout B.

The *Fat Loss Revolution* strength training programs are designed to be performed by doing three workouts per week, alternating between workout A and workout B on non-consecutive days. Each workout program will take approximately 40-45 minutes per workout, excluding the warm up.

Execute the exercises as a pair. Perform one set of A1 and one set of A2. Rest for the time indicated, then do another set of A1 and A2, and rest again. Repeat until you've completed all of the specified sets for the A exercises, and then move on to B1 and B2.

Perform Phase 1 Workouts A and B for four weeks.

After four weeks of Phase 1 Workouts A and B, you will change to a completely new exercise program, Phase 2 Workouts A and B.

After four weeks of Phase 2 Workouts A and B, you will change to another completely new exercise program, Phase 3 Workouts A and B.

Tempo is the speed of movement to perform the exercise that is indicated with a three digit number such as 402. The first number is the eccentric or lowering action of the exercise, the middle number is the pause or isometric hold, and the third number is the concentric of For example, an squat with a tempo of 412 you will lower your body for a count of 4 seconds, hold for one second at the bottom of the squat and return to standing for a count of two seconds. Any exercise with a tempo of XXX is an indication to perform that exercise as fast as possible, with optimal technique, of course.

**"How much weight should I use?"**

The amount of weight (load) to be used for each exercise is not indicated on the *Fat Loss Revolution* programs because you will determine the load based on the number of repetitions specified in each program. The load will be different for each individual. Always master each exercise with your bodyweight before adding additional load or weight.

*Always focus, concentrate and maximize quality over quantity.*

Lighter weights and higher repetitions are recommended during the introductory phase for all individuals who are new to strength training or those without prior experience. New trainees must strengthen their joints, tendons and connective tissue first. From a safety and developmental standpoint, this initial phase encourages a foundation and development of quality motor engrams, ensuring proper exercise technique, injury prevention and quality of movement.

Selecting a weight that is challenging is a key component of the *Fat Loss Revolution* workout programs. As you progress, use a load that is heavy enough to create an optimal training stimulus. The weight you select should allow you to do one or two more reps than the recommended number of reps on the programs. If a specific exercise indicates 10-12 repetitions and you can only get eight with the weight you selected, the weight (load) is too heavy, indicating that you should reduce the weight for the next set. The same concept applies if you are able to get 15-20 reps when the program suggests 10-12 reps; this is an indication that the load is too light and you should use a heavier weight on your next set.

Every single repetition should be performed with perfect technique; i.e., your last rep and first rep should look identical.

---

*Never compromise exercise technique or form.*

---

## Be Smart – Warm Up Properly for the Best Workout

**A dynamic warm up** is performed immediately before the actual workout using active muscular effort to increase body temperature and range of motion without holding the end position. Moving dynamically stimulates the nervous system and prepares your muscles, joints and connective tissue for the upcoming workout. Ideally, it is best to mimic the anticipated movements, activity or exercises that follow your warm up routine.

Once your body is properly warmed up, you will be prepared to perform each exercise with proper technique so you maximize results and minimize risk of injury.

Perform five to ten minutes of dynamic movement and preparatory exercises specific to each workout. Here is an example of some preparatory exercises:

* Jump rope, 200-500 contacts, or 25-30 jumping jacks
* Kettlebell swings
* Forward and lateral band walks (mini-band around the front area of the foot)
* 10-12 body weight squats
* 5 lunges with rotation, right and left
* 5 hip circles, each leg
* 10 forward (pendulum) leg swings, each leg
* 10 side (pendulum) leg swings, each leg
* 10-12 pushups
* 5-10 spiderman crawls

The foam roller can be used both before and after your workout. Exercises for specific muscle groups using the foam roller can be found by visiting my blog, http://thepowerof4-paula.blogspot.com.

## Be Smart – Cool Down

Upon completion of your workout, include static stretching and foam rolling to maximize flexibility and specifically target the fascia. Fascia is a strong, fibrous connective tissue, the most influential structure that affects flexibility.

This is also the perfect time to sip on your post-workout shake.

Foam rolling can be included as part of the warm up as well. However, static stretching is best done immediately following exercise (never before) by holding each stretched position for 20 to 60 seconds. Static stretching is effective for muscle recovery and very calming to the nervous system.

## Phase 1 – Workout A

**Week 1 and Week 3**

Program design instructions (see page 182)

Dynamic warm up (see page 184)

In addition, perform one set of 10 repetitions of exercises A1 and A2 with 50 percent of the weight you plan to use for your first set.

| Order | Exercise | Sets | Reps | Tempo | Rest |
|---|---|---|---|---|---|
| A1 | Underhand lat pulldown | 3 | 10-12 | 402 | 30-60 |
| A2 | Front foot elevated 4" Dumbbell split squat | 3 | 10-12 | 402 | 30-60 |
| B1 | 45° Incline dumbbell chest press (palms facing in) | 3 | 10-12 | 402 | 30-60 |
| B2 | Dumbbell goblet squat | 3 | 12-15 | 303 | 30-60 |
| C1 | Prone dumbbell I-Y-T on 45° incline bench | 3 | 6 ea | 212 | 30-60 |
| C2 | Swiss ball leg curl | 3 | 12-15 | 202 | 30-60 |

Cool down.

## Phase 1 – Workout A

**Week 2 and Week 4**

Program design instructions (see page 182)

Dynamic warm up (see page 184)

In addition, perform one set of 10 repetitions of exercises A1 and A2 with 50 percent of the weight you plan to use for your first set.

| Order | Exercise | Sets | Reps | Tempo | Rest |
|-------|----------|------|------|-------|------|
| A1 | Underhand lat pulldown | 4 | 12,10, 8, 12 | 402 | 45-60 |
| A2 | Front foot elevated 4" Dumbbell split squat | 4 | 12,10, 8, 12 | 312 | 45-60 |
| B1 | 45° Incline dumbbell chest press (palms facing in) | 4 | 12,10, 8, 12 | 402 | 45-60 |
| B2 | Dumbbell goblet squat – wide stance | 4 | 12,10, 8, 12 | 303 | 45-60 |
| C1 | Prone dumbbell I-Y-T on 45° incline bench | 3 | 6 ea | 212 | 30-60 |
| C2 | Swiss ball leg curl | 3 | 12-15 | 201 | 30-60 |

Cool down.

## Phase 1 – Workout A – Illustrations

Underhand Lat PullDown

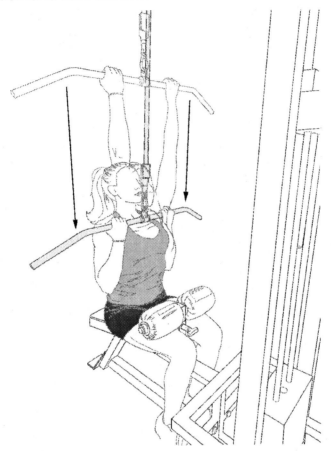

1. Position roller pads so they are in contact with the top of your thighs.

2. With an underhand grip, position your hands on the bar slightly wider than shoulder width.

3. Keeping your torso upright, pull the bar down to your front shoulders and upper chest. Visualize bringing your chest to the bar as you engage the muscles in your back.

4. Slowly straighten your arms and return to the starting position.

## Front Foot Elevated Dumbbell Split Squat

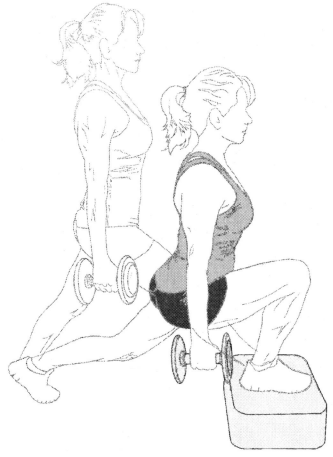

1. Place your right foot on a 4-6 inch platform. With feet hip-width apart, extend your left leg behind you approximately 3 feet.

2. Slowly lower your body until the right hamstring just comes into contact with the right calf. Right knee should track in line with your middle toe. Your knee should not extend forward beyond the toes. Left heel remains lifted.

3. Make sure to distribute the weight evenly on the right foot and drive through the heel as you extend the right leg straight, engaging your quad and glute. Complete all reps on your right leg and switch to the left foot on the step.

## 45° Incline Dumbbell Chest Press

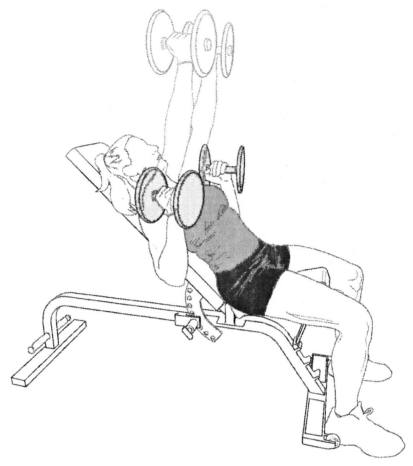

1. Lie face up on a 45° incline bench holding the dumbbells above your shoulders with palms facing one another. Keep feet flat on the floor.

2. Slowly lower the dumbbells to outside your shoulders and upper chest with elbows close to your torso.

3. Press the dumbbells back up to the starting position as you engage your chest muscles.

## Dumbbell Goblet Squat – Option #1

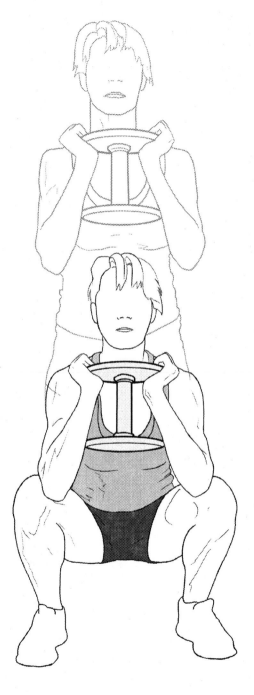

1. Hold a dumbbell vertically at your chest, with both hands cupping the end of the dumbbell.

2. Elbows should point down to the floor.

3. Position feet slightly wider than your hips.

4. Keeping torso upright and abs tight with back naturally arched, squat down until thighs are parallel to the floor or lower. Make sure your knees track in line with the middle toe and keep your heels firmly on the floor.

5. Exhale as you return to starting position while engaging your glutes.

# Dumbbell Goblet Squat – Option #2 Wide Stance

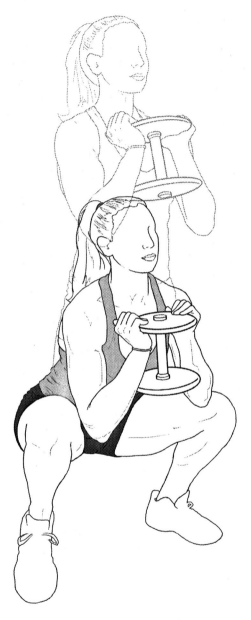

1. Hold a dumbbell vertically at your chest, with both hands cupping the end of the dumbbell.

2. Elbows should point down to the floor.

3. Position feet wider than your hips angling feet at a 10 o'clock and 2 o'clock stance.

4. Keeping torso upright with abs tight and back naturally arched, squat down until thighs are parallel to the floor or lower. Make sure your knees track in line with the middle toe and keep your heels firmly on the floor.

5. Exhale as you return to starting position while engaging your glutes.

## Prone Dumbbell I-Y-T on 45° Incline Bench

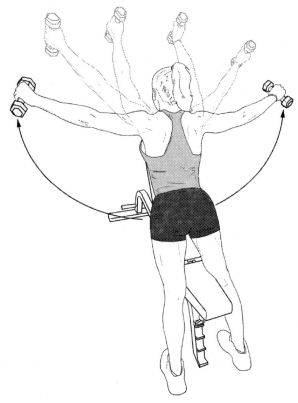

1. Lie face down on a 45° incline bench with dumbbells and your chest at the top of the bench.

2. Keeping abs tight, squeeze glutes and imagine pulling your front ribcage into your back as you keep your chest down on the bench.

3. Maintain a neutral spine with head and neck aligned with shoulder blades back and down.

4. "I" position: with straight arms and palms facing one another, raise the dumbbells so your biceps are next to your ears in a letter "I" position at the top of the movement. Slowly return the weights to starting position. "Y" position: with straight arms and palms facing one another, raise the dumbbells to form a letter "Y" and slowly return the weights to starting position. "T" position: with straight arms, raise the dumbbells to form a letter "T" with palms facing the floor at the top of the movement. Slowly return the weights to the starting position. This constitutes one repetition.

## Swiss Ball Leg Curl

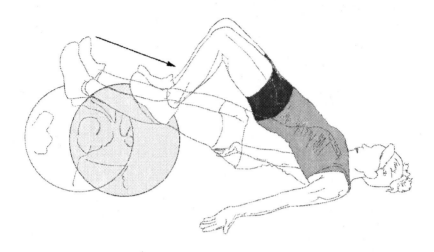

1. Lie on floor with heels on a Swiss ball.

2. With arms at your sides, turn knuckles down so that palms face the ceiling.

3. Raise your hips so your body is in a straight line. Keep your abs tight and engage your glutes.

4. Keeping your hips lifted, drive heels into the ball and bring the ball toward your butt. Make sure feet remain straight up.

5. Reverse the position.

## Phase 1 – Workout B

### Week 1 and Week 3

Program design instructions (see page 182)

Warm up (see page 184)

In addition, perform one to two sets of exercises A1 and A2 with 55 and 65 percent of the weight you plan to use for your first set.

| Order | Exercise | Sets | Reps | Tempo | Rest |
|-------|----------|------|------|-------|------|
| A1 | Romanian deadlift | 3 | 10-12 | 501 | 60 |
| A2 | Standing dumbbell push press | 3 | 10-12 | 201 | 60 |
| B1 | 3-way directional DB lunge (forward, lateral, transverse) | 3 | 6 reps each | 302 | 60 |
| B2 | Standing row to neck with rope (elbows up and out) | 3 | 10-12 | 312 | 60 |
| C1 | Pushups (elevate upper body if needed) | 3 | 10-20 | 201 | 60 |
| C2 | Swiss ball triple threat (straight leg hip extension, leg curl, bent knee hip extension) | 3 | 10 each | 212 | 60 |

Cool down.

## Phase 1 – Workout B

**Week 2 and Week 4**

Program design instructions (see page 182)

Warm up (see page 184)

In addition, perform one to two sets of exercises A1 and A2 with 55 and 65 percent of the weight you plan to use for your first set.

| Order | Exercise | Sets | Reps | Tempo | Rest |
|-------|----------|------|------|-------|------|
| A1 | Romanian deadlift | 4 | 10, 8, 6, 10 | 402 | 60 |
| A2 | Standing dumbbell push press | 4 | 10, 8, 6, 10 | 20X | 60 |
| B1 | Dumbbell stepup (10-14") | 4 | 10, 8, 6, 10 | 202 | 60 |
| B2 | Standing row to neck with rope | 4 | 10, 8, 6, 10 | 312 | 60 |
| C1 | Pushups (elevate upper body if needed) | 2 | 10-20 | 201 | 60 |
| C2 | Hip extension (lie on floor, knees bent, heels on bench) | 2 | 10-20 | 222 | 60 |

Cool down.

## Phase 1 – Workout B – Illustrations

Romanian Deadlift

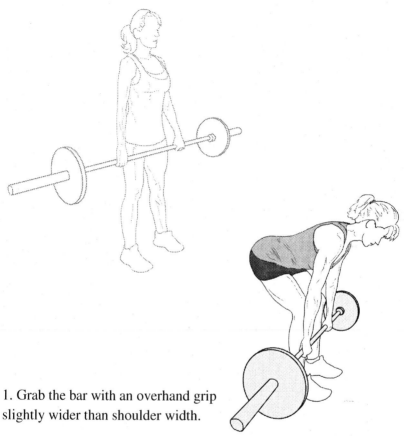

1. Grab the bar with an overhand grip slightly wider than shoulder width.

2. Position feet hip-width apart.

3. Keep abs tight. Maintain alignment of your spine as you initiate the movement from your hips. Bend at your hips pushing them back. Bend your knees approximately 20 degrees. Lower your torso until it is parallel to the floor.

4. The bar stays in close contact with the legs as you return to the starting position engaging your hamstrings and glutes. Keep your head in line with your torso to prevent compression in the neck.

## Standing Dumbbell Push Press

1. Hold a pair of dumbbells at your shoulders with palms facing each other.

2. Bend your knees 20° and drive with your legs as you press the dumbbells overhead.

3. Keep abs tight and front ribs drawn in to prevent compression in the low back when arms press overhead.

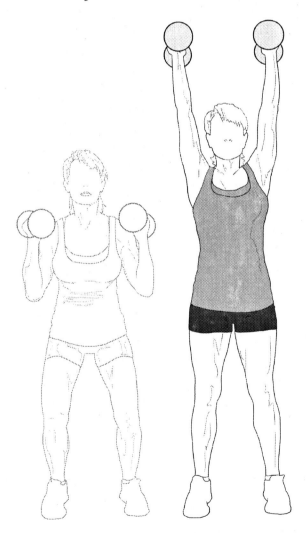

## 3-way Directional Dumbbell Lunge

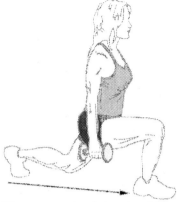

1. Hold a pair of dumbbells. Stand with your feet hip-width apart. Take a step forward with your right leg approximately 2-1/2 to 3 feet as you lunge down until your thigh is parallel to the floor. Your heel should contact the floor first. Lunge down until your thigh is parallel to the floor. Your back leg is almost straight and the knee is two to three inches from the floor. Keep your abs tight, shoulders back and spine aligned.

2. Driving through your right heel, step back to the starting position as you engage the glute muscle.

3. Immediately lunge to the right side as you push your hips back, keeping your torso upright. Both feet should be flat with the toes pointing forward. In the lunge position, the left leg will be straight with the kneecap lifted, engaging the quadriceps muscle.

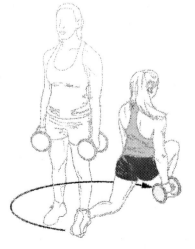

4. Drive through the right foot as you return back to starting position.

5. Immediately rotate 135° to the right and take a step forward into a lunge as you pivot onto the left toe.

6. Keep your torso upright and abs tight as you lunge with the right thigh parallel to the floor.

## Dumbbell Stepup (10-14")

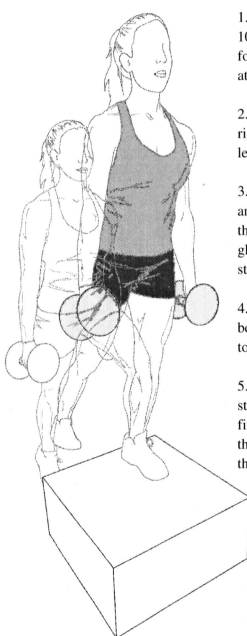

1. Place your left foot on a 10-14" stepup box with the foot turned out just slightly at 5°.

2. Lift your toes up on the right foot and keep the right leg straight.

3. Drive through the left foot and engage the quadriceps of the left leg and squeeze your glutes as the left leg straightens.

4. Keep the left knee aligned between the second and third toe as you slowly step down.

5. Left foot remains on the step until all reps are finished. Finish all reps on the left leg and repeat with the right foot on the step.

## Standing Row to Neck With Rope

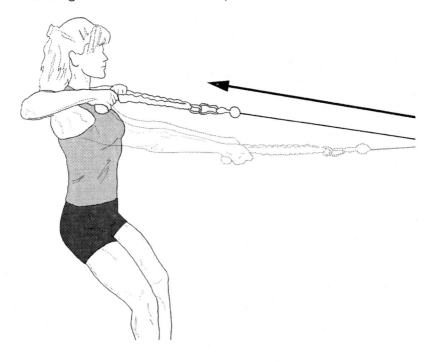

1. Attached a rope to the middle cable of a pulley machine (approximately chest height) and grab the end of the rope in each hand with palms facing one another.

2. Step back until there is tension in the cable with arms straight, feet hip-width apart and knees bent 20 degrees.

3. Keeping your abs tight, pull the rope toward your neck and upper chest area with elbows up and out squeezing your shoulder blades together. Keep front ribs pulled down and in.

4. Slowly extend arms back to starting position.

Pushups

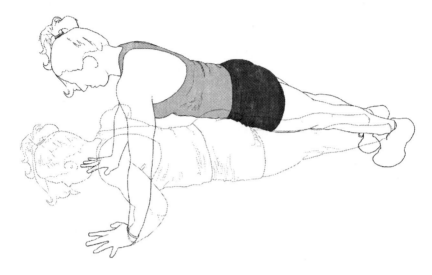

1. Hands slightly wider than shoulder width.

2. Your body should maintain a straight line from your heels to your head. Keep your spine aligned throughout the pushup. Lower your body until your chest nearly touches the floor (bench or bar).

3. Maintain a contraction in the abdominals and squeeze your glutes. Keeping all fingers pressed into the floor, exhale as you push your body up and away from the floor. Engage your upper back muscles at the top of the push up by puffing up your upper back so there is not a dip between the shoulder blades.

To make the pushup easier, elevate your upper body by placing your hands on a bench or bar.

If the traditional pushup is too easy, place your feet onto a bench, Swiss Ball or some other raised surface or lift one leg.

## Swiss Ball Triple Threat

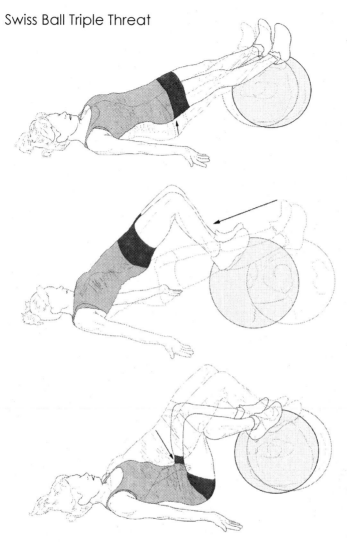

1. Straight leg hip extension – lie on your back with heels on a Swiss Ball and palms face up. Lift hips, pressing heels into the ball, and keep body in a straight line as you squeeze your glutes. Keep feet straight up. Finish all reps and immediately move on to the Swiss ball leg curl.

2. Swiss ball leg curl – see page 194 for instructions. Finish all reps and move on to the bent leg hip extension.

3. Bent leg hip extension – with bent legs, lift and lower hips with feet on the ball.

## Hip Extension

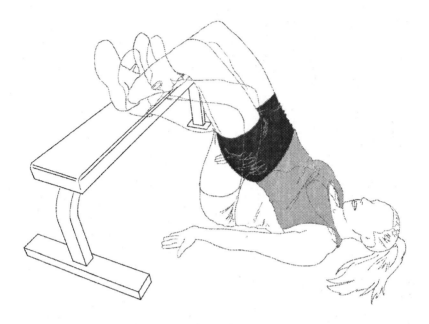

1. Lie on the floor face up with knees bent at a 90° angle with heels on a bench and palms up.

2. Keeping your abdominals braced, squeeze your glutes tightly as you dig your heels into the bench and raise your hips until your body forms a straight line from your shoulders to your knees.

3. Lower your body to the starting position.

## Phase 2 – Workout A

### Week 1 and Week 3

Program design instructions (see page 182)

Dynamic warm up (see page 184)

In addition, perform one to two sets of exercise A1 for 4 reps using the jump stretch band. Perform 1-2 sets of A2 with 55 and 65 percent of the weight you plan to use for your first set.

| Order | Exercise | Sets | Reps | Tempo | Rest |
|-------|----------|------|------|-------|------|
| A1 | Close grip chinup (use jumpstretch bands) | 3 | 4-8 | 501 | 90 |
| A2 | Conventional deadlift | 3 | 8-10 | 401 | 90 |
| B1 | Dumbbell pushup and row | 3 | 12-16 | 202 | 60 |
| B2 | Dumbbell lunges (in place lunge forward, press back) | 3 | 8-12 | 302 | 60 |
| C1 | Swiss ball side flexion, Right side, left side | 3 | 10-15 each side | 202 | 60 |
| C2 | 45° back extension (hinge at hip) | 3 | 10-12 | 202 | 60 |

Cool down.

## Phase 2 – Workout A

### Week 2 and Week 4

Program design instructions (see page 182)

Dynamic warm up (see page 184)

In addition, perform one to two sets of exercise A1 for 3–4 reps using the jump stretch band. Perform one to two sets of A2 with 55 and 65 percent of the weight you plan to use for your first set.

| Order | Exercise | Sets | Reps | Tempo | Rest |
|-------|----------|------|------|-------|------|
| A1 | Close grip chinup (use jumpstretch bands) | 4 | 4-6 | 511 | 90 |
| A2 | Conventional deadlift | 4 | 10,8, 6, 10 | 402 | 90 |
| B1 | Dumbbell pushup and row | 4 | 10-16 | 202 | 60 |
| B2 | Walking dumbbell lunges | 4 | 10,8, 6, 10 | 302 | 90 |
| C1 | Swiss ball pushup and jackknife | 2 | 8-20 | 202 | 60 |
| C2 | 45° back extension (hinge at hip) | 2 | 10-12 | 212 | 60 |

Cool down.

# Phase 2 – Workout A – Illustrations

Close Grip Chinup (assisted using a jumpstretch band)

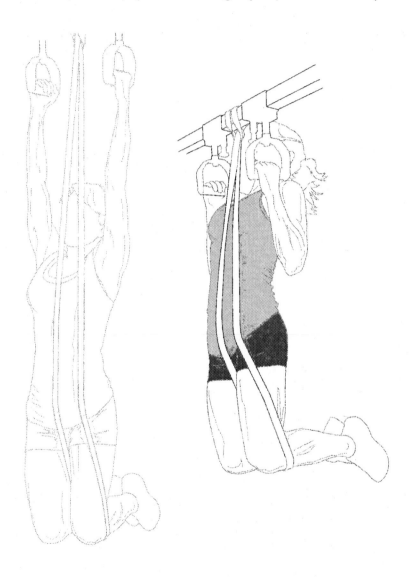

See the next page for instructions.

**Instructions for Close Grip Chinup**
**(assisted using a jumpstretch band)**

1. Loop a jumpstretch band around a chinup bar and pull it through the other end so the band is tightly secure to the bar.

Use a thicker band to make the chinup easier and a thinner band to increase the intensity. You can also use two bands to make the chinup easier.

2. Grab the bar with palms facing one another. Place one or both knees in the loop of the band and hang at arms length.

3. Imagine pulling the bar toward you as you squeeze your shoulder blades down and squeeze your pinky fingers on the bar. Keep knees directly under hips.

4. Pull your chest to the bar until your chin comes to or above the bar.
5. Slowly lower your body until arms are straight and repeat.

Purchase jumpstretch bands at PaulaOwens.com/store.html.

## Conventional Deadlift

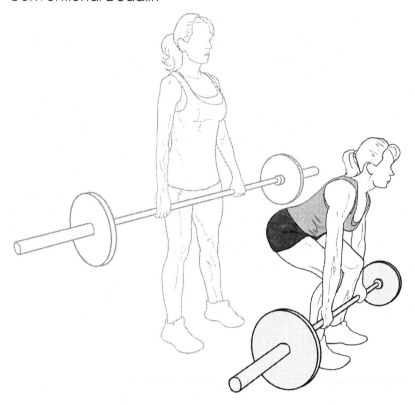

1. Load an Olympic barbell and grab it with an overhand grip slightly wider than your shoulders.

2. Rotate the inside elbow forward.

3. Keeping your arms straight and the bar against your legs with a neutral spine, bend at your hips and knees, pushing your hips back. Low back has a slight lordotic curve, upper and mid-back do not round and head is aligned with torso. In the bottom position, the bar is over shoelaces and torso forms a 45° angle to the floor.

4. Keep your abs tight and strongly drive your feet into the floor as you pull the bar to your knees following through with the hips (activating your hamstrings and glutes) as you return to the starting position.

## Dumbbell Pushup and Row

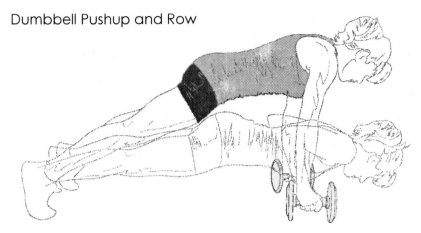

1. Assume a pushup position with a pair of dumbbells and body forming a straight line from your heels to your head.

2. Keeping abs tight and spine neutral, lower your chest toward the floor. Stop a few inches from the floor and push back up.

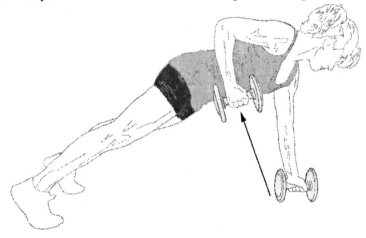

3. At the top of the pushup, row the dumbbell in your right hand to the side of your chest and ribcage without rotating your torso as you stabilize your body on the left arm.

4. On the next pushup, row the dumbbell in the left hand.

5. Continue to alternate right and left until all reps are completed. To make the exercise easier, elevate upper body and omit the dumbbells. To make it harder, place your feet on a raised surface.

## Dumbbell Lunges

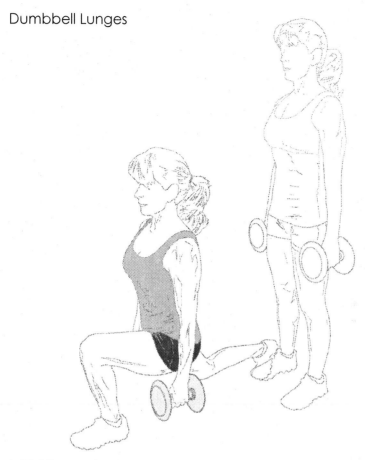

1. Holding a pair of dumbbells or kettlebells at your sides, stand with your feet parallel and hip-width apart.

2. Take a step forward approximately 2-1/2 to 3 feet with your left leg, keeping your back straight and your eyes looking straight ahead. Your left heel should contact the floor first as you step forward and your knee should track over your middle toe. Lunge down until your left thigh is parallel to the floor. Your back leg is nearly straight with the knee two to three inches from the floor and the heel lifted.

3. Keep your abs tight, shoulders back and spine aligned as you drive through your left heel, stepping back to the starting position.

4. Complete all reps on the left leg and switch to the right leg.

## Walking Dumbbell Lunge

1. With feet hip-width apart, take a step forward approximately 2-1/2 to 3 feet long with your right leg. Your heel should contact the floor first.

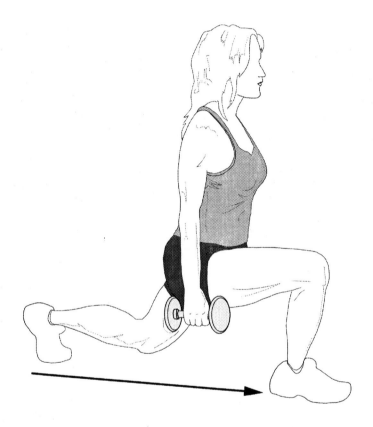

2. Keeping your torso upright, lunge down until your thigh is parallel to the floor. Keep your knee in line with your middle toe. Your back leg is nearly straight as you lunge with the knee two to three inchesfrom the floor.

3. As you rise up from the lunge, immediately step forward with your left leg into a lunge.

4. Continue alternating each leg as you lunge forward, finishing all reps.

## Swiss Ball Side Flexion

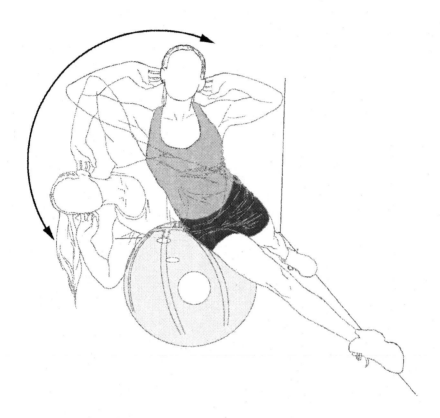

1. Position yourself on your right side on a Swiss ball with your right hip stacked on top of your left hip and bottom leg forward.

2. Bend sideways over the Swiss ball, keeping your abs tight.

3. As you lower your body, armpit comes in contact with Swiss ball.

4. Exhale as you return to the starting position.

5. Finish all reps and repeat on the other side.

## Swiss Ball Push Up and Jackknife

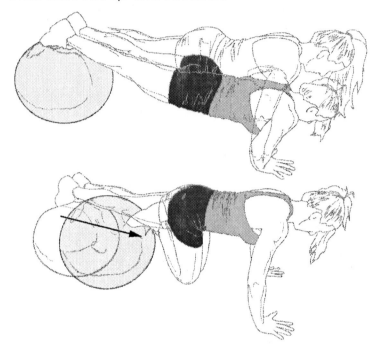

1. Place your feet on a Swiss ball and your hand on the floor slightly wider than shoulder width with index fingers parallel to one another.

2. Keep your abs tight, spine neutral and squeeze your glutes as you lower your body without dropping your hips. At the bottom position, your head will be above your hands (not between your hands).

3. Exhale as you push yourself back up to the starting position.

4. Using your feet, pull the ball in toward your chest without rounding your low back.

5. Keep your abs braced as you return the ball back to the starting position. This is one rep.

6. If you are unable to complete the pushups with optimal technique, be sure to finish all reps for the jackknife (bottom illustration).

## 45° Back Extension

1. Position the pad of the machine so it is at the top of your thighs.

2. Position feet onto platforms with ankles against padding and place hands at ears. (To make the exercise easier, fold arms at chest; to increase intensity, extend arms overhead.)

3. Hinge at hip keeping your abs tight and back and neck neutral.

4. Squeeze your glutes and raise your torso until your body is in a straight line.

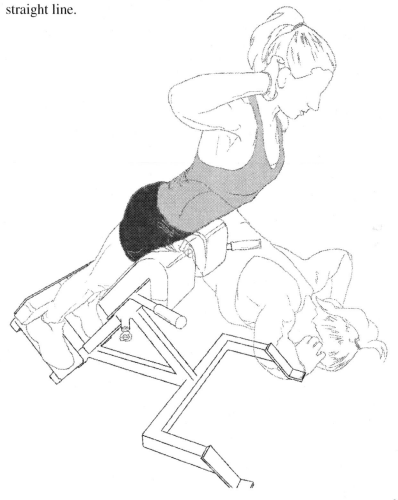

## Phase 2 – Workout B

### Week 1 and Week 3

Program design instructions (see page 182)

Dynamic warm up (see page 184)

In addition, perform one to two sets of exercise A1 for eight to ten reps using 50 and 65 percent of the weight you plan to use for your first set.

Perform one set of exercise A2 for eight reps with the bar elevated higher than the height you plan to place the bar for your first set.

| Order | Exercise | Sets | Reps | Tempo | Rest |
|-------|----------|------|------|-------|------|
| A1 | Barbell or dumbbell squat | 3 | 8-12 | 402 | 60 |
| A2 | Inverted horizontal row (overhand grip) | 3 | 8-12 | 311 | 60 |
| B1 | Dumbbell side step up (10-14") | 3 | 8-12 | 202 | 60 |
| B2 | Single arm low pulley "lawnmower" row | 3 | 8-12 | 301 | 60 |
| C1 | Hip thrust (upper body on bench) | 3 | 12-15 | 222 | 60 |
| C2 | Swiss ball jackknife or pike | 3 | 8-10 ea | 212 | 60 |

Cool down.

## Phase 2 – Workout B

**Week 2 and Week 4**

Program design instructions (see page 182)

Dynamic warm up (see page 184)

In addition, perform one to two sets of exercise A1 for eight to ten reps using 50 and 65 percent of the weight you plan to use for your first set.

Perform one set of exercise A2 for eight reps with the bar elevated higher than the height you plan to place the bar for your first set.

| Order | Exercise | Sets | Reps | Tempo | Rest |
|-------|----------|------|------|-------|------|
| A1 | Barbell front squat | 4 | 8, 6, 6, 8 | 402 | 60 |
| A2 | Inverted horizontal row (underhand grip) | 4 | 8-12 | 312 | 60 |
| B1 | Dumbbell side step up (10-14") | 4 | 8, 6, 6, 12 | 202 | 60 |
| B2 | Single arm low pulley "lawnmower" row | 4 | 8, 6, 6, 12 | 211 | 60 |
| C1 | Hip thrust (upper body on bench) | 2 | 10-12 | 212 | 60 |
| C2 | Swiss ball jackknife or pike | 2 | 10-20 ea | 211 | 60 |

Cool down.

## Phase 2 – Workout B – Illustrations

### Barbell or Dumbbell Squat

1. Hold a bar across your upper back below the seventh vertebrae, the "meaty" area of your upper trapezius muscle. If you are unable to axial load the spine by placing a bar on your upper back due to scoliosis or some other limitation, hold a pair of dumbbells with arms straight at your sides.

2. With feet slightly wider than hip width, position your elbows so they are directly under the bar and keep them there.

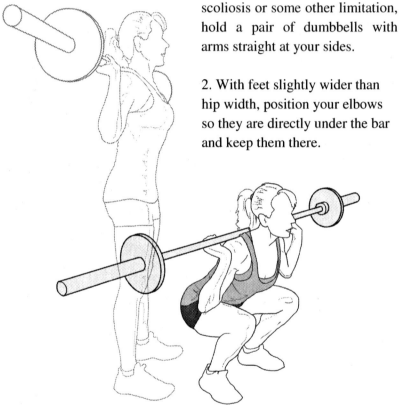

3. Keeping abs tight, spine neutral and torso upright, look forward (not up) as you squat down to parallel or lower without losing the natural arch in your lower back.

4. Knees should track in line with the middle toe and keep your heels firmly on the floor.

5. Exhale as you drive your heels into the floor and return to the starting position.

## Barbell Front Squat

1. With arms crossed, hold a bar on your front shoulders or take an overhand grip on a bar bending your elbows under the bar so that it rests on the front of your shoulders.
2. Feet are slightly wider than hip-width, with toes pointing slightly out.
3. Raise your arms until they are parallel to the floor, with elbows up and pointing straight ahead. Keep them there for the entire set.

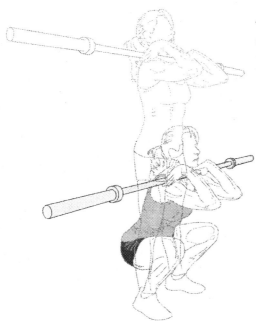

4. Keeping abs tight, spine neutral and torso upright, look forward (not up or down) as you push your hips back, squatting down to at least parallel or lower without losing the natural arch in your lower back.
5. Knees should track in line with the middle toe.
6. Exhale as you drive your feet into the floor and return to the starting position.

## Inverted Horizontal Row

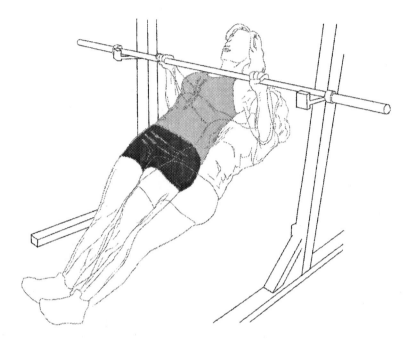

1. Set a bar securely in a squat rack or Smith machine. To determine the height for the bar, you should be able to perform all repetitions on the program with good form. To modify the exercise and make it easier, either raise the bar higher and move your feet back or bend your knees to a 90° angle. To increase difficulty, lower the bar or elevate your feet onto a raised surface or set a weight plate on your chest.

2. Grab the bar with an overhand or underhand grip (as indicated on the exercise program) slightly wider than your shoulders and hang from the bar. It is extremely important that the body remains rigid and in a straight line from your head to your heels with abs engaged throughout the entire exercise.

3. Pull your chest to the bar and pause for a moment at the top.

4. Slowly lower your body back to the starting position.

## Dumbbell Side Stepup

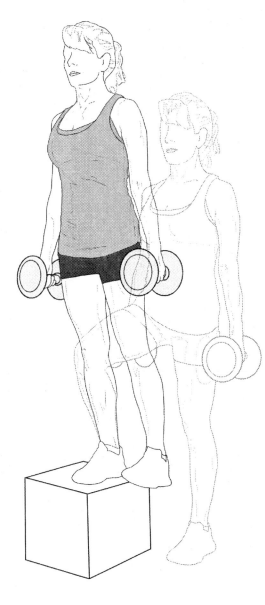

1. Stand at the side of a 10-14" stepup box. Place the right foot onto the step with the foot turned out just slightly at 5°.

2. Drive through the right foot, making sure to keep the heel down. Lift the toes up on the left foot and keep the left leg straight as you step up, straightening the right leg. Engage the quadriceps as the right leg straightens.

3. Keep the right knee aligned between the middle toe and slowly step down.

4. Finish all reps on the right leg and repeat with the left foot on the step.

## Single Arm Low Pulley "Lawnmower" Row

1. Attach a handle to the low pulley and grab the handle with your left hand.

2. Facing the pulley, step back into a staggered split stance with the right foot forward and your left arm straight. Left heel is lifted.

3. Hinge at the hips, reaching forward, and pull the handle to your left side, activating the muscles in your back as you rotate your body to the side. Left foot will rotate and flatten. Keep your abs tight.

4. Straighten your left arm and finish all of the reps on the left side.

5. Switch to the right arm and complete all of the reps.

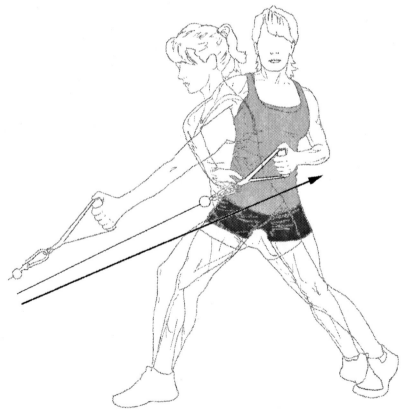

## Hip Thrust

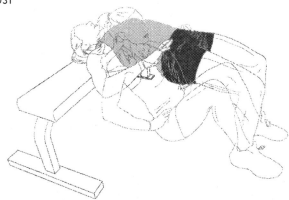

1. Place your mid-to-upper back perpendicular on a flat bench with your butt on the floor and feet hip-width apart.

2. Initiate the movement by using your glutes, pressing your feet into the floor as you thrust your hips up with control. Keep your spine neutral. At the top, your knees will be bent 90° and your body will be in a straight line from your knees to your head. Squeeze your glutes at the top.

3. Once you master the hip thrust with your body weight, you can progress by adding resistance. If you use a barbell, make sure to pad the area of the bar that will be placed on your hips.

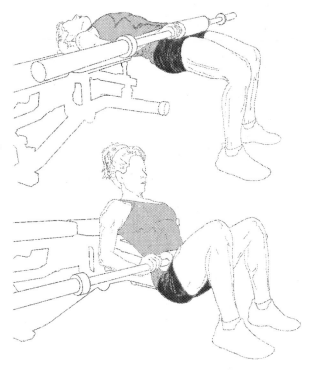

## Swiss Ball Pike

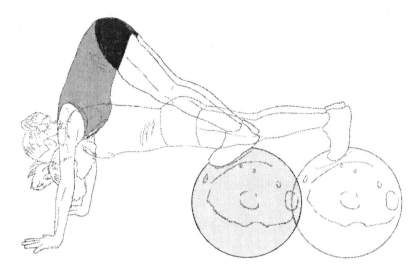

1. Assume pushup position with hands slightly wider than shoulder width and toes on a Swiss ball.

2. Keeping legs straight and abs tight, bend your hips, lifting them into the air into an inverted "V" position as you pull the ball toward your chest.

3. Slowly roll the ball back as you lower your hips to the starting position.

4. To increase intensity, add a pushup after you roll the ball back to starting position.

## Phase 3 – Workout A

### Week 1 and Week 3

Program design instructions (see page 182)

Dynamic warm up (see page 184)

In addition, perform one to two sets of exercise A1 for three to four reps using the jump stretch band. Perform one set of exercise A2 with 55 percent of the weight you plan to use for your first set.

Note for exercise B1: Perform six reps with the incline bench at a 60° angle, immediately lower the bench to 45° for four reps, immediately lower the bench to 30° for four more reps. That's a total of 14 reps for one set.

| Order | Exercise | Sets | Reps | Tempo | Rest |
|-------|----------|------|------|-------|------|
| A1 | Underhand chinup (use jump stretch bands) | 3 | 4-6 | 511 | 60 |
| A2 | Dumbbell split squat | 3 | 8-12 each leg | 312 | 60 |
| B1 | Descending incline dumbbell chest press 60°/45°/ 30° | 3 | 6-4-4 | 302 | 60 |
| B2 | Sumo deadlift | 3 | 8-10 | 302 | 60 |
| C1 | Upper pulley chop, right and left | 3 | 10-12 each side | 201 | 30 |
| C2 | Prone 45° dumbbell lateral raises | 3 | 10-12 | 312 | 30 |

Cool down.

## Phase 3 – Workout A

### Week 2 and Week 4

Program design instructions (see page 182)

Dynamic warm up (see page 184)

In addition, perform one to two sets of exercise A1 for three to four reps using the jump stretch band. Perform one to two sets of A2 with 55 and 65 percent of the weight you plan to use for your first set.

Note for exercise B1: Perform four reps with an incline bench at a 60° angle, immediately lower the bench to 45° for two reps, immediately lower the bench to 30° for two more reps. That's a total of 8 reps for one set.

| Order | Exercise | Sets | Reps | Tempo | Rest |
|-------|----------|------|------|-------|------|
| A1 | Underhand chinup (use jump stretch bands) | 4 | 6, 5, 4, 6 | 401 | 60 |
| A2 | Overhead reverse barbell lunge | 4 | 6-10 each leg | 201 | 60 |
| B1 | Descending incline dumbbell chest press 60°/45°/ 30° | 4 | 4-2-2 | 302 | 60 |
| B2 | Sumo deadlift | 4 | 6-10 | 302 | 60 |
| C1 | Upper pulley chop, right and left | 2 | 10-12 each side | 10X | 30 |
| C2 | Prone 45° dumbbell "Y" raises | 2 | 8-12 | 212 | 30 |

Cool down.

# Phase 3 – Workout A – Illustrations

Underhand Chinup (assisted using jumpstretch band)

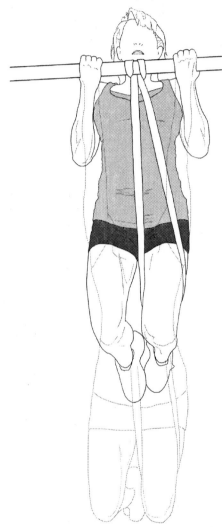

1. Loop a jumpstretch band around a chinup bar and pull it through the other end so the band is tightly secured to the bar. Use a thicker band to make the chinup easier and a thinner band to increase the intensity.

2. Grab the bar with a shoulder-width underhand grip. Place one or both knees in the loop of the band and hang at arms length.

3. Imagine pulling the bar toward you as you squeeze your shoulder blades down and squeeze your pinky fingers on the bar. Keep knees directly under hips.

4. Pull your chest to the bar until your chin comes to or above the bar.

5. Slowly lower your body until arms are straight and repeat. Progressively challenge yourself using thinner jumpstretch bands to eventually perform the chin up unassisted and with your body weight.

Purchase jumpstretch bands at PaulaOwens.com/store.html.

## Dumbbell Split Squat

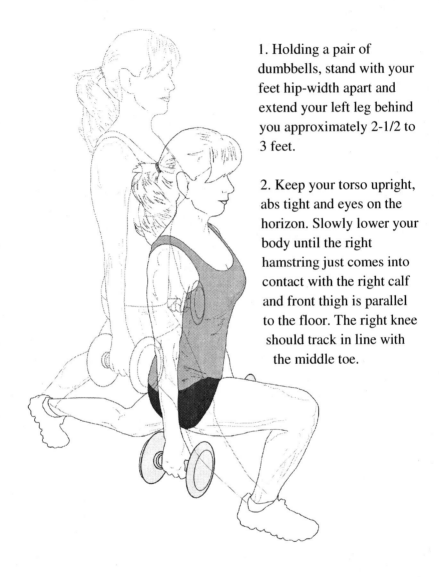

1. Holding a pair of dumbbells, stand with your feet hip-width apart and extend your left leg behind you approximately 2-1/2 to 3 feet.

2. Keep your torso upright, abs tight and eyes on the horizon. Slowly lower your body until the right hamstring just comes into contact with the right calf and front thigh is parallel to the floor. The right knee should track in line with the middle toe.

3. Make sure to distribute the weight evenly on the right foot, keeping the right heel firmly into the floor. Drive through the right foot as you extend your right leg straight, engaging your quad and glute as you return to the start position.

4. Complete all reps on your right leg and switch to the left leg.

## Overhead Reverse Barbell Lunge

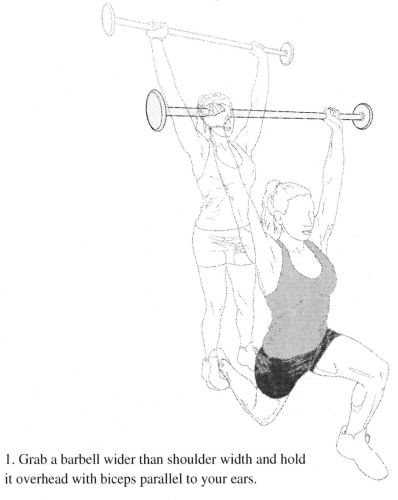

1. Grab a barbell wider than shoulder width and hold it overhead with biceps parallel to your ears.

2. Lunge backwards with your right leg. Left thigh should be parallel to the floor.

3. Keep your arms straight and shoulders down from your ears. Abs remain tight and front rib cage is pulled in with chest lifted.

4. Driving through the left foot, return the right foot to the starting position.

5. Finish all reps on the right side. Switch to the left leg lunging back.

# Descending Incline Dumbbell Chest Press

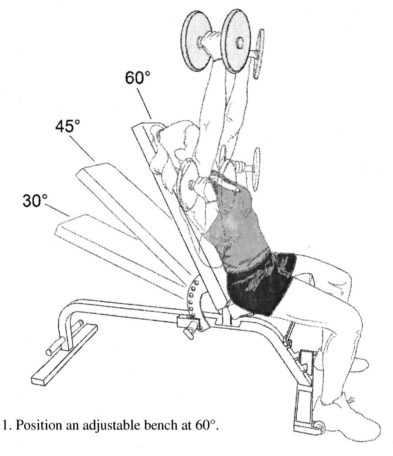

1. Position an adjustable bench at 60°.

2. Lying face up, hold the dumbbells in the
middle of each handle with a semi-supinated (palms face in) grip.

3. With dumbbells overhead, slowly lower them to the shoulder and
outer chest area and then press the weights back up.

4. Continue for the number of reps indicated on the program and
immediately lower the bench to 45° and do the number of reps
indicated.

5. Immediately lower the bench to 30° and do the remaining reps.
This equals one set.

## Sumo Deadlift

1. Grip a barbell with a mixed-grip (overhand grip and underhand grip), placing your hands approximately 12 inches apart.

2. Position your feet wider than your hips, angling your feet at a 10 o'clock and 2 o'clock stance.

3. Keeping your spine neutral and abs tight, bend the hips and knees as you lower your body.

4. Drive your feet into the floor as you thrust your hips forward and straighten your legs, engaging your inner thighs and your glutes.

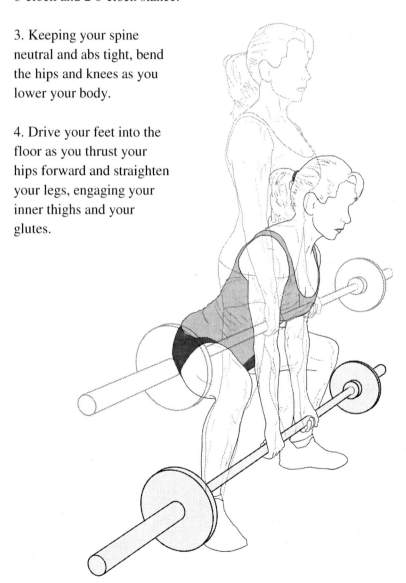

## Upper Pulley Chop

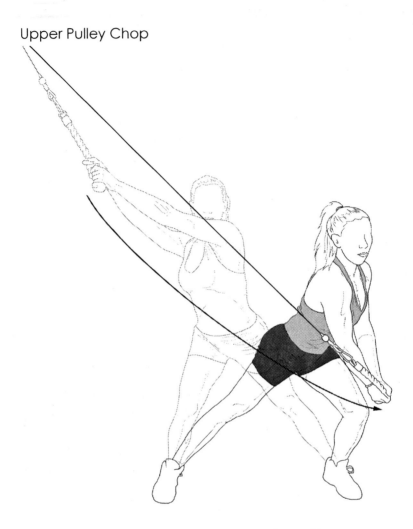

1. Attach a rope to the upper pulley of a cable machine.

2. Grab the rope with both hands and stand to the side of the pulley with a wide stance.

3. Keeping arms straight, pull the rope down to outside thigh as you shift your weight, bending the knee.

4. As you return to start position, opposite knee bends.

5. Finish all reps and continue to other side to complete the set.

## 45° Prone Dumbbell Lateral Raises

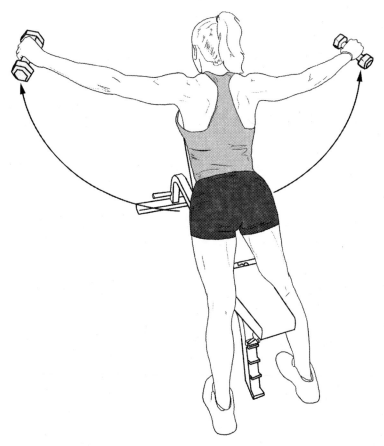

1. Lie face down on a 45° incline bench with dumbbells.

2. Keeping abs tight, squeeze glutes and imagine pulling your front ribcage into your back body as you keep your chest down on the bench.

3. Maintain a neutral spine with neck aligned with shoulder blades back and down.

4. With a soft elbow, raise the dumbbells so they are in line with your ears at the top position.

5. Slowly return weights to starting position.

## 45° Prone Dumbbell "Y" Raises

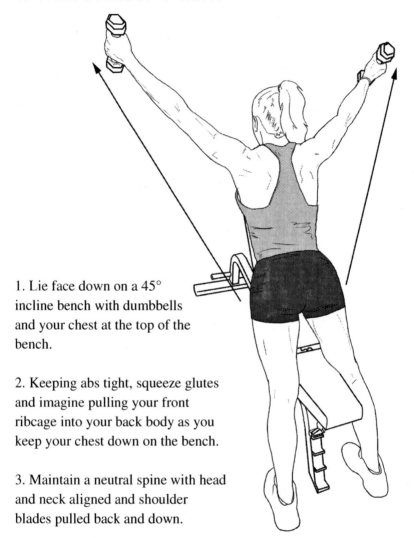

1. Lie face down on a 45° incline bench with dumbbells and your chest at the top of the bench.

2. Keeping abs tight, squeeze glutes and imagine pulling your front ribcage into your back body as you keep your chest down on the bench.

3. Maintain a neutral spine with head and neck aligned and shoulder blades pulled back and down.

4. With straight arms and palms facing one another, focus on using the rear shoulders and raise the dumbbells to form a letter "Y." Pause at the top of the movement as you engage your rhomboids, the muscles between your shoulder blades.

5. Slowly return the weights to starting position.

# Phase 3 – Workout B

## Week 1 and Week 3

Dynamic warm up (see page 184)

In addition, perform two sets of exercises A1 and A2 with 55 and 65 percent of the weight you plan to use for your first set.

Note for exercise B1: Perform six reps, immediately get four more reps with a lighter weight, immediately get four remaining reps with an even lighter weight. That's a total of 14 reps for one set.

| Order | Exercise | Sets | Reps | Tempo | Rest |
|-------|----------|------|------|-------|------|
| A1 | Single arm dumbbell snatch | 3 | 8-10 | 11X | 30 |
| A2 | Split squat with single arm dumbbell shoulder push press | 3 | 10-12 | 201 | 30 |
| B1 | Flat dumbbell chest press (palms face one another) | 3 | 6-4-4 | 302 | 30 |
| B2 | Bulgarian dumbbell split squat | 3 | 8-12 | 303 | 30 |
| C | Low pulley scarecrow | 3 | 8-10 | 212 | 30 |

## Finisher – Leg Circuits

Perform one to three sets of the following leg circuit exercises as fast as possible using a tempo of **XXX** with proper form and technique.

| | | |
|---|---|---|
| Prisoner Squats | 20 reps | immediately move to ↓ |
| Alternating Lunges | 10 each leg | immediately move to ↓ |
| Power Plyo Lunges | 10 each leg | immediately move to ↓ |
| Squat Jump | 10 reps | Rest 90 seconds |

Cool down.

## Phase 3 – Workout B

**Week 2 and Week 4**

Dynamic warm up (see page 184)

In addition, perform two sets of exercises A1 and A2 with 55 and 65 percent of the weight you plan to use for your first set.

Note for exercise B1: Perform four reps, immediately get four more reps with a lighter weight, immediately get four remaining reps with an even lighter weight. That's a total of 12 reps for one set.

| Order | Exercise | Sets | Reps | Tempo | Rest |
|---|---|---|---|---|---|
| A1 | Single arm dumbbell snatch | 4 | 8, 6, 6, 10 | 11X | 60 |
| A2 | Split squat with single arm dumbbell shoulder push press | 4 | 8, 6, 6, 10 | 201 | 60 |
| B1 | Flat dumbbell chest press (palms face one another) | 3 | 4-4-4 | 302 | 60 |
| B2 | Bulgarian dumbbell split squat | 3 | 4-4-4 | 312 | 60 |
| C | Low pulley scarecrow | 2 | 10-12 | 211 | 30 |

**Finisher – Leg Circuits**

Perform one to three sets of the following leg circuit exercises as fast as possible using a tempo of XXX with proper form and technique.

| | | |
|---|---|---|
| Prisoner Squats | 20 reps | immediately move to ↓ |
| Alternating Lunges | 10 each leg | immediately move to ↓ |
| Power Plyo Lunges | 10 each leg | immediately move to ↓ |
| Squat Jump | 10 reps | Rest 90 seconds |

Cool down.

# Phase 3 – Workout B – Illustrations

## Single Arm Dumbbell Snatch

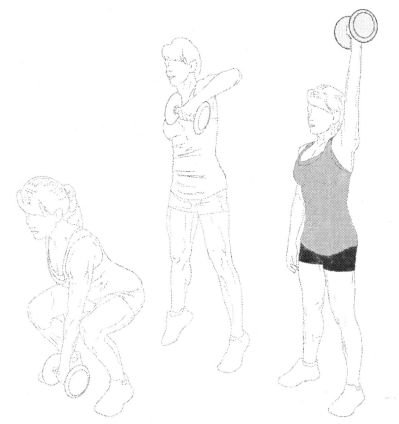

1. Grab one dumbbell. With feet slightly wider than your hips, squat down with the dumbbell centered between your legs.

2. Keeping the dumbbell close to your body, pull the dumbbell straight up to your chest as fast as you can with the elbow high and pointing to the ceiling, coming onto your toes as your legs straighten.

3. Immediately flip and rotate the dumbbell straight up overhead as fast as possible as you straighten your arm and legs.

4. With control, lower the dumbbell back to starting position. Finish all reps on the left arm before switching to the right.

## Split Squat With Single Arm Dumbbell Push Press

1. Hold a dumbbell in the right hand, standing with feet hip-width and step the right foot back into a split squat position. Feet should be hip width, not on a straight line as though standing on a tightrope.

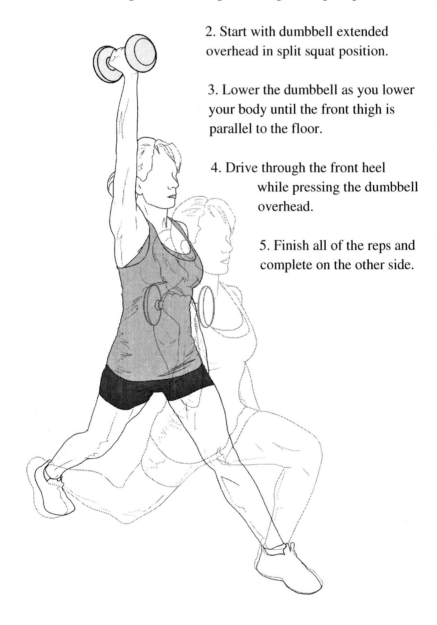

2. Start with dumbbell extended overhead in split squat position.

3. Lower the dumbbell as you lower your body until the front thigh is parallel to the floor.

4. Drive through the front heel while pressing the dumbbell overhead.

5. Finish all of the reps and complete on the other side.

## Flat Dumbbell Chest Press

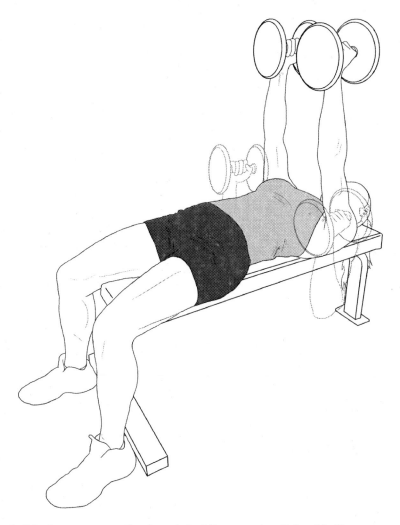

1. Lie face up on a flat bench holding a pair of dumbbells over your chest with a semi-supinated (palms facing in) grip and feet flat on the floor.

2. Keeping the front ribs pulled down, slowly lower dumbbells to the sides of upper chest.

3. Press the dumbbells back up to starting position, exhaling and engaging the chest muscles.

## Bulgarian Dumbbell Split Squat

1. With feet hip-width apart, stand approximately 3 feet in front of a bench. Keeping your right foot on the floor, place your left foot on the bench behind you. Hold a pair of dumbbells in your hands.

2. Slowly lower your body so your right knee is bent to 90°, thigh is parallel to the floor and your left knee comes close to touching the floor. Your right knee should track in line with your middle toe. The Bulgarian split squat uses the rear leg only for balance as the forward leg does the majority of the work.

3. Your torso should remain upright and abs tight. You should feel a stretch in your rear leg hip flexor and quad as you descend.

4. Push yourself back to starting position by driving your right foot into the floor as you straighten your leg and engage your right glute.

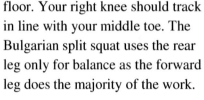

5. Finish all reps on the right leg and switch legs.

## Low Pulley Scarecrow

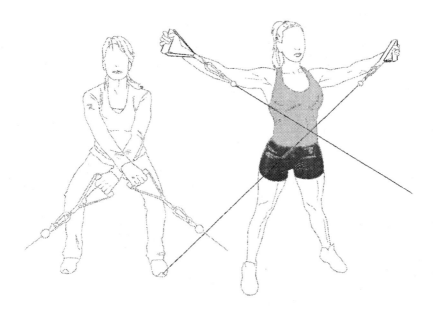

1. Attach a handle to the low pulley of each side of a cable machine.

2. Stand in the middle of the pulleys and grab the right handle with your left hand and the left handle with your right hand so the handles are crossed.

3. Bend legs approximately 20°, keeping spine neutral. Arms will maintain a slight bend (soft bend) at the elbow.

4. Straighten your legs as you pull the handles up and across your body, initiating the movement from the upper back and rear shoulder area.

5 At the top of the movement, knuckles should be in line with your ears.

6. Lower the handles to the starting position.

# Leg Circuits – Body Weight

Perform the four leg circuit exercises as fast as possible.

## Prisoner Squats

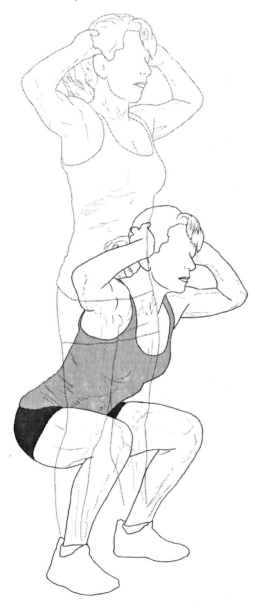

1. Stand with feet slightly wider than hip-width. Place hands on head next to ears.

2. Keeping your abs tight, spine neutral and eyes on the horizon, squat down to at least parallel. Knees should track in line with middle toes.

3. Imagine as though you are pushing the floor away as you drive your feet into the floor and return to starting position as fast as possible.

Perform the reps for the prisoner squat as fast as you can with perfect technique.

## Alternating Lunges

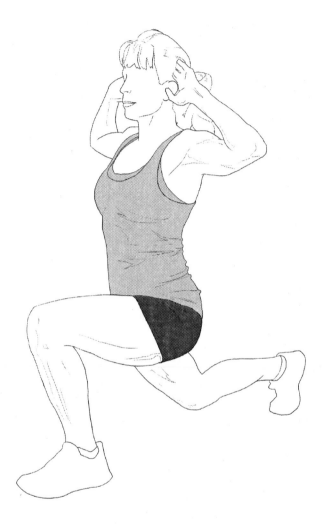

1. Stand with feet hip-width apart. With hands at the side your head at the ears, lunge forward, alternating between right and left legs as fast as possible.

2. Keep abs tight and torso erect. Knee tracks in line with middle toe.

3. Drive and push through the front heel as you lunge forward and step back.

## Plyometric Lunges

Plyometric lunges should be performed as fast as possible.

1. Standing with feet hip-width apart, lunge forward approximately two to three feet with your right leg.

2. Keep your torso upright as you swing your arms overhead to give you more air height. Explosively jump straight up as high as you can so both feet leave the floor and switch legs while in the air.

3. Land softly and lightly with your left leg forward.

4. With minimal time on the ground, immediately jump back up as you continue to alternate legs.

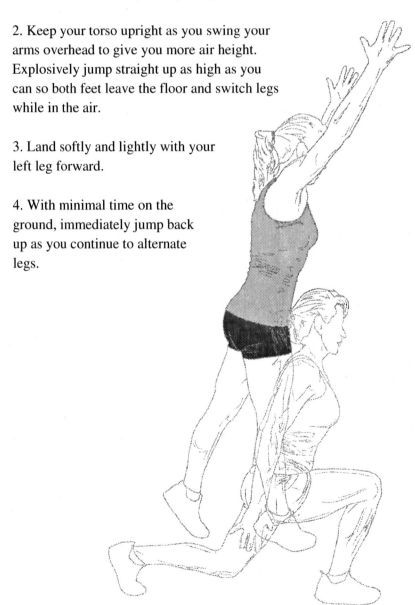

## Squat Jump

The squat jump should be performed as fast as possible with a narrow or wider stance.

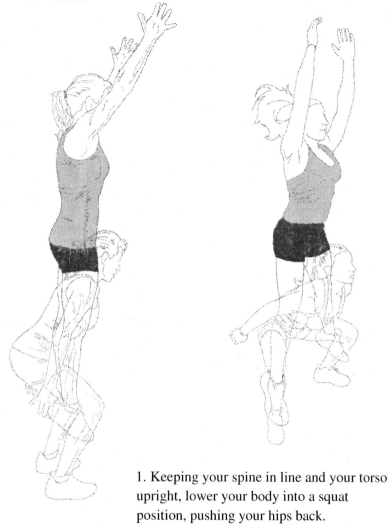

1. Keeping your spine in line and your torso upright, lower your body into a squat position, pushing your hips back.

2. Explosively jump straight up as high as you can. Swing your arms overhead to give you more air.

3. Land softly and lightly, and immediately squat down and jump up explosively again. Keep knees in line over the middle toes.

## Interval Fat Blaster – Rev It Up for a Hot 'n Healthy Body

The REV workouts are fast-paced, intense, time-efficient workouts that focus on density – the total amount of work done in a specific length of time.

There are two different REV workouts: REV Workout #1 and REV Workout #2. Perform one of the REV workouts one day per week, and perform the other REV workout the following week, alternating between the two workouts.

After completion of the REV workouts, your metabolism will be revved up for up to 36 hours after completion of the workout.

The REV workouts are perfect for when you're pressed for time. The exercises in the REV workouts target all of the major muscle groups and are performed with short rest intervals.

The REV workouts are highly effective and will increase muscle, improve aerobic and anaerobic capacity, maximize hormonal response and promote fat loss – the perfect combination to achieve a hot 'n healthy body.

Be sure to record your REV workout progress in your workout journal.

*Never compromise exercise technique or form.*

## REV It Up – Workout #1

The exercises in REV Workout #1 will be performed in a circuit-style fashion for a specific length of time.

◈_____◈

**Level 1** (Level 1 is anyone who is embarking on a new exercise program or who has never exercised.)

Perform as many repetitions as possible for each exercise in a 20-second time frame. Take 20 seconds of rest and move on to the next exercise. Repeat until you have completed all of the exercises on the program. Listen to your body. Initially, you may need a longer rest period between exercises. After the last exercise on the workout, rest for two to three minutes. Repeat the complete circuit two times.

◈_____◈

**Level 2** (Level 2 is for an intermediate level or seasoned exerciser who has been exercising consistently for at least two years.)

Perform as many repetitions as possible of each exercise in a 30-second time frame. Take 30 seconds of rest and move on to the next exercise. Continue to the next exercise. After the last exercise on the workout, rest for two minutes. Repeat the complete circuit two to four times.

◈_____◈

Keep track of your progress. Count the number of repetitions you achieved for each exercise and record them in your workout journal every time you perform the REV workouts.

*Your last repetition should look identical to your first repetition.*

## Dynamic warm up for the REV workouts

Using a medicine ball, perform the following exercises for 12-15 repetitions each (*see illustrations*).

A1      Squat push press

A2      Swing through and extend

A3      Torso twist

A4      Diagonal woodchop


**REV workout program #1** *(see illustrations)*

A1      Single arm dumbbell or kettlebell swing

A2      Pushups

A3      Squat thrust (burpees)

A4      Prisoner speed squats (hands on head at ears)

A5      Medicine ball slams

A6      Squat jumps or jumping jacks

A7      Mountain climbers


Cool down.

## REV It Up – Dynamic Warm Up – Illustrations

Squat Push Press With Medicine Ball

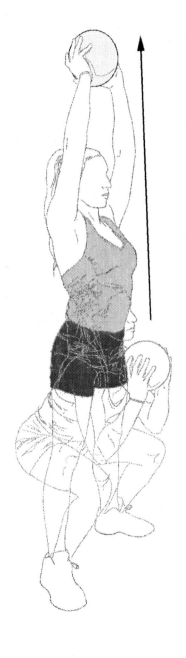

1. Hold medicine ball at chest, in squat position. Elbows contact top of thighs. Feet are positioned at 1 o'clock and 11 o'clock.

2. In squat position, knees should align between second and third toes. Avoid knees dropping in.

3. Extend up from the squat into standing position, driving through heels as you press the ball overhead. Biceps will be in line with the ears when the ball is overhead. Keep front ribs pulled in to prevent compression in the low back.

## Swing Through and Extend With Medicine Ball

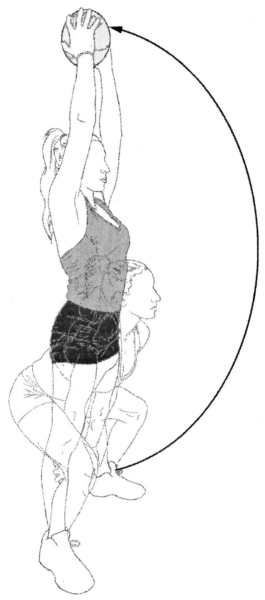

1. Holding medicine ball over head, lower into squat position, taking medicine ball through legs.

2. Extend up into standing position, driving with hips as you swing the medicine ball overhead.

## Torso Twist With Medicine Ball

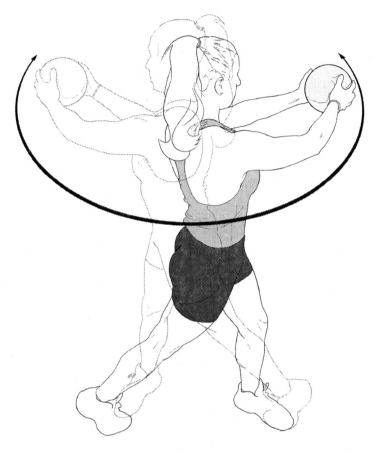

1. Arms are extended in front of chest holding medicine ball. With soft knees, twist right and left with ball at chest level, then waist level, then hip level. Twist back up from hip level, waist, and chest for recommended repetitions. Do not collapse your rib cage.

2. Pivot on the toe during the twisting movement as indicated in the illustration.

## Medicine Ball Diagonal Woodchop

1. Keeping eyes focused on
the medicine ball and arms
straight, pivot on left toe,
rotating torso to the right
and bringing medicine
ball to outside of calf.

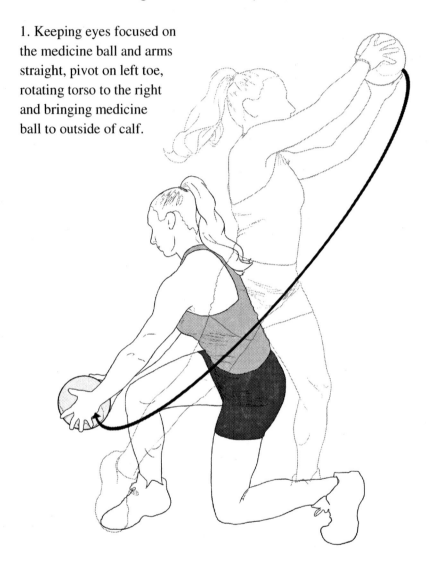

2. Using a diagonal chopping motion, rotate torso to the left, pivoting
on right toe and bringing medicine ball overhead to the left.

3. Finish 12 to 15 reps and repeat on other side.

## REV Workout #1 – Illustrations

Single Arm Kettlebell or Dumbbell Swing

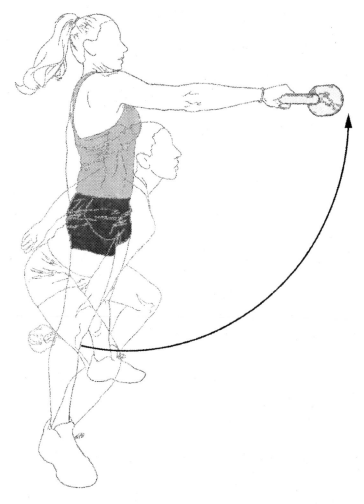

1. Keeping your arm straight, swing the kettlebell somewhat forcefully through your legs.

2. Thrust your hips forward as you extend to standing position, bringing kettlebell to chest level.

3. Repeat with other arm.

## Pushup

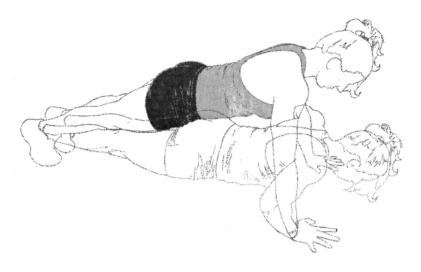

1. Place hands slightly wider than shoulder width.

2. Your body should maintain a straight line with your spine aligned throughout the pushup. Lower your body until your chest nearly touches the floor (bench or bar).

3. Maintain a contraction in your abdominals and squeeze the glutes. Keeping all fingers pressed into the floor, exhale as you push your body up and away from the floor. Engage your upper back muscles at the top of the pushup by puffing up your upper back so there is not a dip between the shoulder blades.

If you're unable to perform a pushup on the floor, elevate your upper body so your hands are on a bench or bar.

If the traditional pushup is too easy, elevate feet onto a bench or Swiss Ball, or lift one leg.

## Squat Thrust

Perform as fast as possible.

1. Squat down, placing hands on the floor.

2. Jump back into a pushup position.

To increase intensity, add a pushup.

3. Jump feet back toward hands.

4. Jump up explosively.

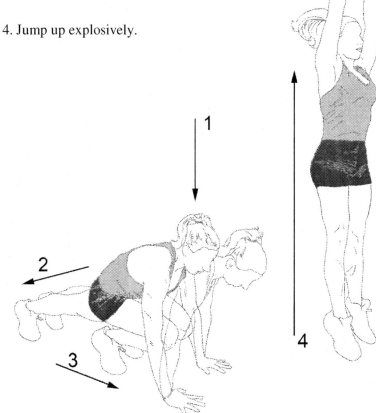

## Prisoner Speed Squat

Perform the reps as fast as you can with perfect technique.

1. Stand with feet slightly wider than hip-width. Place hands on head next to ears.

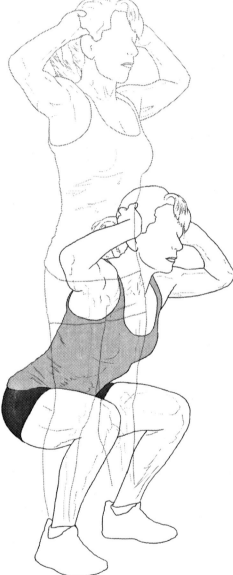

2. Keeping your abs tight, spine neutral and eyes on the horizon, squat down to at least parallel. Knees should track in line with middle toes.

3. Imagine as though you are pushing the floor away as you drive your feet into the floor and return to starting position as fast as possible.

## Medicine Ball Slam

1. Explosively slam the medicine ball from above your head to the floor continually for the recommended number of repetitions or number of seconds indicated on the program.

2. Keep your abs tight and spine neutral.

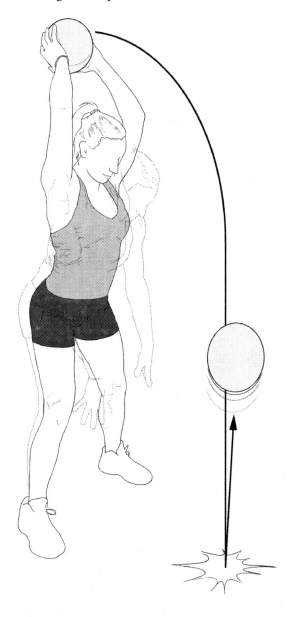

## Squat Jump

Perform as fast as possible.

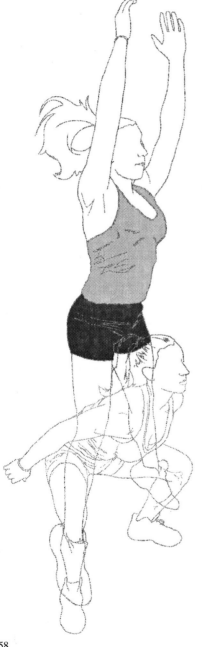

1. Keeping back straight, lower your body into a squat position until thighs are parallel to the floor.

2. Explosively jump up as high as you can, using your arms for height.

3. Land softly and lightly and immediately squat down and jump up again. Keep knees in line over middle toes.

4. The squat jump can also be performed with a narrower stance with feet hip-width (see page 245).

## Mountain Climbers

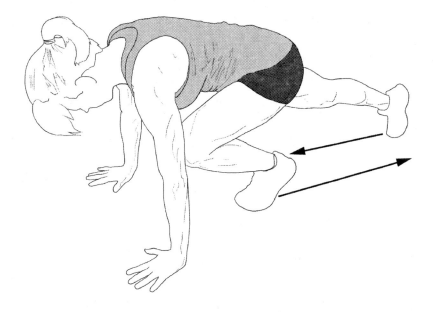

1. Assume a pushup position with hands slightly wider than shoulder width. Imagine as though you are pushing the floor away with your hands.

2. Lifting your left foot, draw your knee as close to your chest as you possibly can without raising your hips into the air.

3. Return your left foot to the starting position, and immediately switch to the right side.

4. Keep abs tight throughout the entire set as you quickly alternate left and right sides.

## REV It Up – Workout program #2

REV Workout #2 is an effective, time-efficient workout perfect for those days when you're short on time. The exercises are split into two segments – Segment A and Segment B. The total length of time for this workout is 15 minutes.

In segment A, alternate between two exercises, A1 and A2, for a total of 12 minutes, resting as needed. It is extremely important that you perform each repetition with perfect form and technique. Focus on quality of movement. Your last repetition should look identical to your first repetition.

In segment B, rotate through three exercises, B1, B2 and B3, for a total of three minutes. Strive to get as many sets as possible in three minutes. Your goal is to perform as many reps as possible during each set with optimal exercise technique and form.

Keep track of your progress. Count the number of repetitions and the amount of weight used for each exercise. Record this information in your workout journal every time you perform the workouts.

## REV It Up – Workout #2 – Select Your Level (1 or 2)

**Level 1** (pertains to anyone who is embarking on a new exercise program or who has never exercised.)

**Segment A exercises:** Perform six to eight repetitions alternating between A1 and A2. Select a weight you can successfully lift for 12-15 reps; this is the weight to be used for A1 and A2. If needed, increase the length of rest between A1 and A2 so that you can complete six to eight reps.

**Segment B exercises:** Rotate through exercises B1, B2, and B3 for a total of three minutes. Do your best and make every effort to get as many reps as you can with optimal form.

Listen to your body. Initially, you may need a longer rest period.

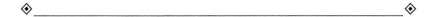

**Level 2** (applies to an intermediate level or seasoned exerciser who has been exercising consistently for at least two years.)

**Segment A exercises:** Perform four to six repetitions, alternating between A1 and A2. You will use a weight that you can lift for eight to ten reps. Increase your rest if needed to complete four to six reps.

**Segment B exercises:** Rotate through exercises B1, B2, and B3 for a total of three minutes, doing your best and making every effort to get as many reps as you can.

Listen to your body. Initially, you may need a longer rest period.

## REV It Up – Workout #2

Dynamic warm up (see page 184)

In addition, perform one set of six to eight repetitions of exercises A1 and A2, with 50 percent of the weight you plan to use for your first set.

See illustrations for exercise description and instructions.

| Order | Exercise | Reps | | Total time |
|-------|----------|------|------|------------|
| | | Level 1 | Level 2 | |
| A1 | Deadlift | 6-8 | 4-6 | 12 minutes |
| A2 | Dumbbell push press | 6-8 | 4-6 | |
| B1 | Pushups | Perform as many reps as possible | | 3 minutes |
| B2 | Inverted row | | | |
| B3 | Lunges | | | |

Cool down.

## Sprint for a Hot 'n Healthy Body at Any Age

The most effective workouts for losing body fat are strength training and high-intensity intervals. With sprint intervals, you will lose body fat, improve your level of conditioning faster and save time. A 2008 study published in the *Journal of Physiology* reported that four to six 30-second sprint intervals produced MORE fat oxidation than 45-60 minutes of moderate intensity cardio.

Another study in the August 2012 issue of *International Journal of Sport Nutrition and Exercise Metabolism* revealed that two minutes of sprinting is equivalent to 30 minutes of jogging. This study found that the significant amount of body fat loss that occurs with sprinting is partially due to the increased metabolism post-workout.

A 2012 study in the *Journal of Obesity* found that men lost four pounds of visceral belly fat in only 12 weeks by sprinting. The subjects sprinted for eight seconds followed by a 12-second recovery phase for a total of 20 minutes, three times a week.

**In just 12 weeks, you can expect these benefits from the *Fat Loss Revolution* sprint workout Rx:**

* Greater amount of fat burned in less time than LSD exercise
* Stronger and leaner legs and hips
* Tighter and more defined abs
* Natural increase in growth hormone
* Elevated metabolism
* Increased anaerobic and aerobic capacity that is far greater than LSD exercise
* Enhanced feelings of well-being
* Lower cortisol and insulin levels
* Increased lean muscle tissue

## Sprint for success

The *Fat Loss Revolution* sprint workouts are intense, mentally challenging, and will deliver profound results when done consistently. Increase your speed and frequency gradually. It is important that you do not go overboard. Less is more when it comes to sprinting. You will achieve the best results when you focus on and maximize quality (intensity) as opposed to quantity (duration).

## Frequency

Perform the sprint workout at least once per week up to three times per week maximum on non-consecutive days. Most people do well with two days per weeks on the days in between their *Fat Loss Revolution* strength training programs. Each person is unique as to what is best for their body.

## Intensity

Perform your sprints with all out, maximum effort, whatever that is for you personally.

If you're a novice to sprinting, an important factor to keep in mind is to start with shorter distances and gradually increase the distance over time. In addition, if this is your first time for this type of workout, take longer periods of active rest. As you become better adapted and conditioned, you can manipulate the length of rest. *Always listen to your body.*

## Variables

If you are unable to sprint outdoors on a rubber track, other options may include a treadmill, spinning bike, stationary bike, rowing machine, stairs, bleachers or an elliptical trainer.

## Ready – Set – It's Time to Sprint

### Dynamic Warm Up
Perform five to ten minutes of movement specific to sprinting. Examples include: Leg swings (front and side), lunge walk with rotation, hip circles, lateral lunges, forward and lateral band walks, alternate iron cross, butt kicks, power skips and dynamic calf movement (see page 184). As part of the warm up, include a 60 percent gradual build-up sprint.

### Sprint Options
Select one of the sprint options below. After a thorough warm up, perform your first set. Rest for the length of time indicated and perform your next set. Active rest can consist of a stroll or slow walk. Repeat until all sets have been completed.

| Length of sprint | Sets | Active rest |
|---|---|---|
| 35 meter | 6-10 | 60-90 seconds |
| 8 seconds | 8-12 | 15 seconds |
| 15 second | 6 | 60 seconds |
| 30 second | 6 | 90 seconds |
| 100 meter | 6-10 | 90 seconds |
| 150 meter | 6 | 2 minutes |
| 200 meter | 6 | 4 minutes |

## More Sprint Options

| Length of sprint | Sets | Active rest |
|---|---|---|
| 60 seconds | 6-8 | 120 seconds |

For this option, find a hill at your local park or an area with an inclined street or sidewalk.

| | | |
|---|---|---|
| 30-60 second hill sprints | 6-8 | 2 minutes |

For this option, visit your local park, beach, high school, community college or any college campus that has bleachers or stairs. If you are traveling, use the staircase in the hotel.

| | | |
|---|---|---|
| 20-30 steps stadiums or stairs | 12-15 | Run up, walk down |

## Cool Down

Static stretching and myofascial release exercises using the foam roller. Exercises for specific muscle groups using the foam roller can be found by visiting my blog:

www.thepowerof4-paula.blogspot.com

*Interval training, especially sprints, will melt your muffin top, flatten your abs and maximize fat loss with dramatically shorter workout sessions.*

# Rest – Relax – Recover – Restore
# for a Hot 'n Healthy Body

A well-rounded, intelligent exercise program includes rest, relaxation, recovery and restoration. Many individuals neglect or disregard the importance of this valuable component for optimal health, strength gains and fat loss. Failure to do so places an incredible strain on the adrenal glands and nervous system and can lead to overtraining.

Balance the more aggressive activities such as sprinting and the *Fat Loss Revolution* strength training programs with rest days, recovery methods and relaxation-type activities. This is necessary for physiological and psychological recuperation, tissue repair and to restore muscle function. The most important muscle recovery is adequate sleep.

Massage, reflexology, ice, gentle stretching and other recovery methods will help reduce stress and tension, minimize inflammation and calm the nervous system. Recovery and relaxation style activities may include yoga, Tai Chi, Qi Gong, golf, deep breathing, meditation or static stretching.

Meditation is the integration of your mind and body with a connection to your soul. During meditation, there is a focused attention on breathing to open up the paths of communication between your body and your brain by quieting the mind. Your breath is the life force. Although the traditional aim of meditation is to increase wisdom, compassion and awareness, meditation can also be used as a method to reduce stress.

Meditation can be integrated during leisurely walking, sitting or while practicing yoga. Remember to breathe fully and deeply.

Regular yoga practice is an excellent complement to the *Fat Loss Revolution* sprint and strength training programs. Yoga encourages flexibility, muscle and organ strength, a composed mind and good health.

Yin yoga is a very passive-style activity that is parasympathetic-based and focuses on lengthening and releasing the fascia, a structure of fibrous connective tissue that surrounds muscles, groups of muscles, blood vessels and nerves. Various asanas (yoga poses) help balance hidden weaknesses, prevent injury and reduce chronic back pain. Overall well-being is enhanced not only on a physical level, but mentally, emotionally and spiritually as well.

Aside from the physical benefits, yoga also provides benefits for the nervous system and the hormonal system. A consistent yoga practice creates a healing power outside of the actual practice itself in which transformation of the mind takes place.

Yoga is a powerful, natural therapy for many diseases and health conditions that can dramatically shift any unhealthy, unsupportive emotions into constructive, encouraging and positive emotions. Yoga releases energetic blockages called *granthis*. These are knots that form at the navel region, the seat of personal power; the heart center, the seat of the emotional body; and the throat, the seat of self-expression. When these blockages are released, physical and emotional layers open up and energy flows freely. This energy, called *prana*, is the essential life-force of all beings.

Deepak Chopra says:

> Any reason for practicing yoga is a good reason. Enhancing flexibility and releasing stress are as noble a purpose for performing yoga as the awakening of spirituality. Yoga serves and nourishes us at every level of our being and spontaneously contributes to greater well-being in all domains of life. Yoga will help you discover gifts within yourself that have remained unopened since your childhood – gifts of peace, harmony, laughter and love.

Honor your body with quiet moments and treat yourself to some form of restoration, relaxation and deep breathing. Rest is essential to hormonal balance (reducing cortisol), tissue regeneration and fat loss.

## Walk This Way for a Hot 'n Healthy Body

Walking is a fabulous lower intensity form of exercise that can be done just about anywhere. Research reports that a brisk, one hour daily walk lessens the genetic influence toward obesity by 50 percent. Simply walking leisurely is an excellent method of recovery and highly beneficial for lowering stress and decreasing cortisol levels.

What I really love about walking is that it:
* can be done outdoors in nature.
* has a minimal risk of injury.
* is relaxing and easy to do.
* is the perfect time to meditate.
* is a powerful activity for reducing stress.
* improves insulin sensitivity.
* helps lower cortisol levels.
* is beneficial for weight control.
* is an excellent recovery activity.
* offers endless benefits to overall health and the mind.
* is free.

Refer to *Chapter 5* for more Stress-less solutions for rest, relaxation, recovery and restoration.

*Walking does the mind and body good, especially when done in nature!*

# CHAPTER 12

## NUTRITIONAL SUPPORT AND SUPPLEMENTS FOR A
## HOT 'N HEALTHY BODY

D o you really need to take supplements? A common belief of many individuals is, "I eat a balanced diet, so I don't need to take vitamins." This statement may have been true back when our grandparents were growing up, but not so in 2012. Ahhh, the good old days, cows actually grazed on grass, chickens were free to roam and lived outdoors, and vegetables were grown in pesticide-free, nutrient-rich soils.

Today's food supply is void of the adequate nutrients required to replenish our body's depleted cells. In addition, every human being is exposed to radiation from cell phones, WiFi, computers and x-rays. Add to that the environmental chemicals from plastics, phthalates, pesticides, herbicides, GMOs and additives, and you have toxic overload.

Unless someone is growing their own vegetables in a nutrient-rich garden, has their own farm with grass-fed cows and free-range chickens and a toxic-free fish pond, it is impossible to obtain all of the required nutrients from food.

Nutrient supplementation is necessary simply because the foods today are lacking in so many vital nutrients. Supplementation will support your biochemistry and help balance the key systems in your body. Therefore, everyone, even the most health-conscious individuals, will benefit from taking high-quality supplements.

## Reasons to add support and protection with nutritional supplementation

* Poor quality agriculture
* Mineral-depleted soils
* Lack of quality in the food supply
* Environmental toxins and pollution
* Unhealthy diet habits
* Prescription and OTC drug use deplete nutrients
* Absorption defects and issues
* Highly processed foods
* Stressful lifestyles
* Recovering from an illness
* Personal nutrient deficiencies

More than 90 percent of individuals are deficient in at least one, if not more, micronutrients. Micronutrients are vitamins, minerals and essential fatty acids. Micronutrient deficiencies are different for each individual and are the cause of a host of symptoms, including headaches, insomnia, depression, thyroid dysfunction, cravings, lack of luster in your hair or skin, low energy, excess weight and many others. Deficiency in any specific nutrient increases the likelihood of being overweight or obese by 80 percent. A study published in the *International Journal of Obesity* found that women who took a daily multivitamin and mineral supplement lost an average of eight pounds compared to 0.5 pounds for the placebo group.

"Biochemical individuality," a term coined by nutritional biochemist Roger Williams, Ph.D., refers to the fact that different people require different nutrients based on their unique genetic make-up.

Nutrition is not a one-size-fits-all plan. Biochemical individuality implies that the amount of each nutrient varies considerably due to individual factors.

Every person has different needs depending on the following:

| | |
|---|---|
| * health status | * previous health history |
| * age | * early dietary habits |
| * metabolism | * biochemical individuality |
| * genetics | * health conditions |
| * physical activity level | * pregnancy |
| * overall lifestyle | * emotional and physical stress |
| * exposure to environmental pollutants and toxins | |

To determine, recommend and provide guidance for a supplement protocol that is specific to your individual requirements and biochemistry, it is important to work with a qualified health care practitioner who is trained in natural therapies and nutrition.

With the mass amount of information and misinformation from the media and the supplement companies, it can be overwhelming to determine the ideal supplements that are most beneficial for you.

Working with a qualified practitioner is not only safer, it is more effective. Harry Eidenier, Jr., Ph.D., states that "supplements should only be purchased from licensed/degreed and trained health care providers and professionals who have the education and clinical experience to provide you with practical information and reliable, non-toxic products."

Many individuals take herbs, vitamins and supplements without knowing or understanding what they're actually taking. For instance, men and post-menopausal women should *not* supplement with a multivitamin that contains iron. Excess iron actually works as a powerful oxidant, increasing free radicals and your risk of cancer.

Only high-quality supplements provide your cells with the best nutrition for health, function and performance. Each person must become an avid label reader and examine the list of ingredients.

Research the brand you buy and the company that owns and makes the brand.

Quality supplements are easier for your body to absorb than most vitamins found in health food stores, supermarkets or discount stores. Poor quality supplements may be harmful to you and hinder health due to the added artificial sweeteners, dyes, coloring, additives, cheap binders, flow agents and fillers.

Quality control is relatively limited in the supplement and vitamin industry. Studies show the body treats synthetic brands, such as those found at large discount warehouses and many health food stores, just like toxic xenobiotics (foreign substances).

It is important that your protein powder, vitamins and other supplements come from a reputable manufacturer and are free of harmful additives, fillers, flow agents and binders, and have undergone a vigorous quality control process.

Licensed or certified practitioners with a degree in nutrition (e.g., naturopaths, chiropractors and nutritionists) are more likely to know which companies are high-quality and which formulas are superior. Ask your health care professional or nutritionist which supplements they personally take. Get your supplements from reliable sources and give your body what it needs!

The wise saying, "You get what you pay for," is certainly true when it comes to vitamins, supplements and protein powder.

> *Supplements are not a substitute for a poor diet.*

## Supplements for a Hot 'n Healthy Body at Any Age

### Primary essentials – the basics

1. Digestzymes (a blend of hydrochloric acid and enzymes specific for digestion)
   - ✓ 2 capsules in the middle of each meal
2. Vitamin D – Bio D Mulsion Forte, an emulsified vitamin D ideal for those with absorption issues
   - ✓ 2 drops at dinner. Test your vitamin D status periodically.
3. Essential fatty acids – EFA Sirt Supreme (fish oil blend of EPA, DHA and GLA)
   - ✓ 3 capsules at breakfast and 3 capsules at dinner
4. BioDoph-7 Plus (Prebiotic)
   - ✓ 1 capsule upon rising
5. 20-14 Pro Flora (whole food probiotic)
   - ✓ 1 capsule 30-60 minutes before bedtime
6. Magnesium glycinate
   - ✓ Start with 400 mg. up to 1000 mg. 30-60 minutes before bedtime
7. Multi-vitamin/mineral taken at breakfast and dinner

According to a study by the University of Aberdeen presented at the British Science Festival, researchers found that after 12 weeks of resistance exercise training, those taking fish oil improved their muscle strength by 20 percent compared with an 11 percent increase in the placebo group.

> *"Always remember to take 800-1000 IU of vitamin E, preferably in the form of mixed tocopherols, whenever you take supplemental oils (fish oils) of any sort. Vitamin E prevents the oil from oxidizing, or becoming rancid too quickly. It also helps your body metabolize the oil effectively."* ~ Jonathan Wright, M.D.

## Secondary – optional

1. Coenzyme Q10
2. Curcumin – Meriva SR
3. L-Carnitine tartrate
4. L-Glutamine
5. Branched chain amino acids (BCAA powder)
6. Antioxidants: Pure Cell; Vitamins C and E

## More supplements for a Hot 'n Healthy Body

* Protein Powders: Vital Whey, Whey Cool or Protein Plus (30-40 gm. after exercise or in a smoothie)
* Detox Powders: NutriClear, Mediclear SGS or Protoclear
* Greens: Greens First, NitroGreens or Women's +40 Greens
* Fiber powders (soluble-rich)
* Green tea and green tea extract

*For a detailed description of the above supplements, visit my online store at PaulaOwens.com*

# CHAPTER 13

## EAT AND DRINK SMARTER FOR A HOT 'N HEALTHY BODY

S imply changing your food choices will have a tremendous impact on the outcome of your overall health and fat loss results. A preference for quality, nutrient-rich foods will sustain your energy, eliminate cravings, balance your mood, provide a feeling of satiety, stabilize blood sugar and fuel your body to induce strength, increase lean tissue and release fat. When you eat more nutrient-rich foods, your cravings disappear and the desire to eat sugary, processed and packaged foods void of nutrients will dissipate.

In this chapter, you will find the *Fat Loss Revolution* "power" foods and beverages to include in your diet to lower your body fat and increase your metabolically-active tissue, prevent or reverse disease, perform better, increase cognitive function, look younger and live longer.

> *"If it doesn't swim, run or fly, or isn't green or growing in the ground, don't eat it."* ~ Charles Poliquin

**Protein** (meaning "of primary importance" in Greek) plays a crucial role in weight control, mood, blood sugar management and your ability to lose body fat. The body does not store protein; hence the need for protein at every meal.

Protein is involved in numerous physiological processes, including building lean muscle, supporting the immune system and maintaining nitrogen balance. Consuming adequate protein will prevent blood sugar fluctuations, increase energy, fuel the brain and eliminate cravings.

Protein is rich in amino acids, which help balance brain chemistry by boosting the levels of mood-regulating neurotransmitters. The first 40 grams of protein you eat every day goes to rebuild your immune system. If you are not rebuilding your immune system, you'll have a hard time rebuilding your brain chemistry to be happy and think straight.

High-protein foods promote thermogenesis (fat burning) and greater satiety than high-carbohydrate, low-fat foods. Animal protein has a three times greater thermic effect than carbohydrates or fat.

In a study published in the *American Journal of Clinical Nutrition,* women on a higher protein diet lost more weight than those eating a carbohydrate diet of the same caloric content. Another study conducted in Sweden revealed that increasing protein intake can reduce weight faster than limiting carbohydrate consumption. Moreover, protein-rich meals tend to make people more alert than sugar or carbohydrate-rich meals.

Numerous studies have shown that a diet with a low carbohydrate to protein ratio and at least 100 grams of protein per day increases fat loss and helps maintain muscle during dieting.

To help you determine how much protein you are actually consuming, here are some guidelines:
* One egg has six grams of protein
* Three ounces of animal protein is equivalent to the size of a deck of cards, which is approximately 20-25 grams of protein.
* Most fish fillets or steaks are about 22 grams of protein for 3 1/2 oz (100 grams) of cooked fish, or 6 grams per ounce.

World-renowned Olympic coach Charles Poliquin recommends that females should eat 40-50 grams of protein before lunch, and males should eat 60-70 grams of protein before lunch.

Some of my personal protein favorites include organic, grass-fed bison, buffalo and beef; whey protein; free-range poultry and pastured eggs; sardines with the bones; wild salmon and other fresh seafood.

**Organic, grass-fed bison, buffalo and beef.** Grass-fed beef is one of richest sources of complete protein, containing all 22 amino acids, including the eight essential amino acids that must be supplied in our diet.

A review in the *Nutrition Journal* reports that organic, grass-fed meats are high in vitamins, antioxidants and omega-3 fatty acids, and loaded with CLA, a healthy fat that boosts immune function, maintains cholesterol and reduces risk of diabetes and cancer. CLA increases metabolism, helping improve body composition. According to the *International Journal of Obesity*, CLA is beneficial in reducing visceral fat. Another study conducted at the University of Wisconsin-Madison reveals that just three grams per day of CLA significantly lowers body fat.

The high-quality protein content in red meat supports muscle retention during weight loss. Grass-fed meats contain many nutrients that can satisfy your appetite so you eat less, stop your body from storing fat and promote thermogenesis. When you eat grass-fed meat, your body is nourished, you are satisfied and the hunger disappears. (See page 103 for more health benefits of including grass-fed beef in your diet.)

**Fish and seafood** have a complete amino acid profile, which is necessary for optimal immune function and cellular repair. Fish is an excellent, nutrient-rich source of protein that contains healthy fats and vitamins A and D. Several types of fish also contain important minerals such as iodine, selenium, potassium and iron.

Individuals who consume fish three to four times a week experience a wide range of health benefits, including better eye and skin health, improved brain function, a healthier functioning heart and an increased ability to manage weight.

Wild salmon (not farmed) is an excellent source of long chain omega-3 fatty acids. Six ounces of wild salmon provides 34 grams of protein. These fatty acids are especially valuable for those who are exercising because of their anti-inflammatory properties.

Depending on where it is caught or raised, or how it is processed, some seafood can be contaminated with chemicals, mercury, PCBs and toxins that can cause serious health problems. Avoid farmed and imported fish.

According to Food & Water Watch, a non-profit organization that works to ensure that the food, water and fish we consume is safe, accessible and sustainable, the "Dirty Dozen" fish (frankenfish) to avoid are:
* Atlantic cod
* Atlantic flat fish (Atlantic halibut, flounder, sole, etc.)
* Caviar
* Chilean seabass
* Eel
* Farmed salmon (Atlantic salmon)
* Imported basa/swa/tra (these are often called catfish)
* Imported farmed shrimp and imported farmed crab
* Orange roughy, shark and Atlantic bluefin tuna

**Free-range poultry.** The term free-range means that the chicken or turkey had access to the outdoors, rather than spending its entire life in a cage the size of a sheet of paper. Free-range poultry is a high-quality source of protein rich in amino acids. Chickens and turkeys raised organically have been fed an organic feed – feed raised without the use of chemical fertilizers or pesticides – for their entire lives and they have never been injected with hormones or antibiotics.

Chickens raised organically actually taste better because of their access to the outdoors, which encourages movement and muscle growth and discourages fat accumulation, and means a leaner, meatier, healthier chicken.

**Eggs** are a nutrient-dense food abundant in vitamins, minerals, essential fats and protein that provide energy and keep you full, while also helping you maintain your muscle as you work to burn away your unwanted fat. Research published in the *International Journal of Obesity* found those who ate eggs at breakfast felt more energetic, snacked less and ate less food at their next meal.

Many individuals dispose of the yolk and eat the egg white only due to their fear of fat and cholesterol. Cholesterol is required for hormone production and many other functions. The egg yolk is the most nutritious part of the egg. The egg yolk contains 43 percent of the total egg protein and has the highest concentration of nutrients, such as amino acids required for optimal brain function, essential fatty acids and vitamins A, E, D, and K. These fat-soluble vitamins support your thyroid, reduce the damaging effects of diabetes; boost your metabolism and immune system; reduce your risk of cancer; encourage healthy bones, teeth and skin; and help you feel fuller longer.

Consuming whole eggs has a positive effect on your appearance and enhances your hair and nails due to the high amount of sulfur, essential fats, vitamins and minerals found in eggs.

Enjoy your eggs sunny side up, over-easy, soft-boiled, hard-boiled, poached or raw. Eggs should be heated lightly and never overcooked to minimize oxidation. When breaking the yolks to scramble eggs, they are exposed to air and heat more than any other cooking method that leave the yolk intact, which causes the fat in the egg yolks to oxidize before you eat them.

Be choosy about where your eggs come from. Avoid omega-3 eggs, which come from chickens that are fed poor-quality sources of omega-3 fats that are already oxidized. Instead, opt for organic, free-range, pastured-raised eggs. Pastured-raised eggs come from chickens that feed on grass and insects, and contain a vast amount of quality nutrients versus eggs from confined chickens.

Eggs from pasture-raised hens have three times more vitamin E, seven times more beta-carotene, two times more omega-3 fats and four to six times the amount of vitamin D as opposed to conventional, factory-farmed eggs.

**Whey protein** is a highly digestible, concentrated protein source full of amino acids. It is high in the amino acid leucine, which helps preserve muscle and promote fat loss. Whey is a powerful antioxidant and an antibacterial that offers immune-enhancing benefits, aids in exercise performance and helps improve body composition.

A study published in the *Journal of the American Dietetic Association* showed that women who supplemented their diets with whey protein lost weight without losing muscle mass. Another study found that whey protein reduces appetite, as well as visceral and subcutaneous fat.

Whey protein stimulates thermogenesis (fat burning) and satiety far greater than casein and soy. Adding whey protein to your diet helps to improve blood pressure cholesterol, lowers insulin levels and increases insulin sensitivity, which has a great impact on body composition.

Remember, not all whey protein is alike. Be sure your protein powders are those that are non-denatured, minimally processed and come only from grass-fed cows without added hormones, steroids or antibiotics. (*See page 176 for more on whey protein.*)

**Vegetarian protein.** For my vegetarian friends, rice, pea or hemp protein powders are alternatives to whey protein.

Hempseed protein is an excellent source of protein that contains all 20 amino acids used in the human body, including all eight essential amino acids. Hemp is also free of oligosaccharides, the component that can cause gas and upset stomach.

Pea protein may be a great choice for individuals wanting to pursue a vegan lifestyle and need extra protein in their diets or for the individual who has a true allergy to milk proteins.

Rice protein is derived by carefully isolating the protein from brown rice. It is a complete protein containing all essential amino acids and nonessential amino acids. Rice protein is hypoallergenic, which makes it suitable for everyone.

Protein powders such as Pure Lean, Peatein or Protein Plus are healthy vegetarian protein alternatives. Vegetarian protein powders should be organic, non-GMO and gluten-free.

Vegan-friendly foods that contain protein include beans, legumes, lentils, nuts, seeds, hemp and chia seeds. Although the combination of rice with beans or legumes is a prominent feature in vegetarian diets, the lectins present in legumes are not well tolerated by many people (lectin intolerance). Many others have grain sensitivities, especially to gluten, or to grain proteins in general.

Vegetarians tend to experience a bit of a challenge burning body fat and building lean tissue without the use of supplemental amino acids, specifically carnitine, carnosine and taurine. In addition to amino acid deficiencies, the majority of vegetarians are often deficient in zinc, hydrochloric acid (HCL), omega-3 fatty acids and vitamins B6, B9 and B12.

**Healthy fats** are necessary for hormone production, healthy skin and hair, heart health, lowering inflammation and encouraging fat loss. Eating foods that are high in fat will not make you fat and eating low-fat or non-fat food will not give you a Hot 'n Healthy Body. Research shows that individuals who consume healthy fats in their diets are leaner and have less body fat. Include more of these healthy fats in your diet: coconuts and virgin coconut oil; olives; cold-pressed, unheated walnut and nut oils; butter; avocado; raw nuts and seeds; organic, pastured egg yolks; grass-fed meats; non-toxic fish and extra virgin olive oil.

**Olive oil** is best used cold since it oxidizes when heated. Extra-virgin olive oil is ideal for drizzling over salads, veggies or fish. Here is a tip to determine if your olive oil is pure, quality olive oil: real olive oil should solidify and thicken after you've stored it in the refrigerator.

**Unrefined coconut oil** is a healthy saturated fat unusually rich in medium chain fatty acids (MCFAs), lauric, caprylic and capric acids. Caprylic acid is an effective and potent antifungal and antimicrobial, which is very helpful for those suffering from Candida, athlete's foot or fungal infections.

Coconut oil is an immune modulator and promotes mitochondrial function (cellular energy). This unique oil promotes lipid oxidation (burns fat), increases metabolism and helps eliminate cravings. A study published in the 2009 *Lipids* journal reported that women who consumed two tablespoons of coconut oil daily over a 12-week period experienced a reduction in waist circumference and an increase in HDL cholesterol. MCFAs found in coconut oil help reverse obesity, resulting in steady weight loss for obese individuals and weight maintenance for healthy people.

In addition, the MCFAs in coconut oil provide an abundance of health benefits, including blood sugar stabilization and thyroid support, and aids in digestive health. The MCFAs do not require emulsification by the liver or the gallbladder. Coconut oil is also nourishing for the brain and improves cognitive function. The metabolizing MCFAs create ketones, which are known to stall or even reverse neurodegenerative diseases such as Alzheimer's.

Coconut oil is the best and safest oil to cook with because it does not oxidize at high temperatures and is resistant to rancidity. Look for organic, unrefined, virgin coconut oil with no other ingredients listed.

**Other healthy oils and fats** include ghee (clarified butter); pastured butter from grass-fed sources; avocado oil; red palm oil; sesame seed oil; macadamia nut oil; and cold-pressed, unheated walnut oil.

**Chia seeds and flax seeds** are a healthy plant source of omega-3 fatty acids that are high in protein and a rich source of fiber. Consumption promotes a feeling of satiety, so you'll naturally eat less. Sprinkle chia seeds or freshly ground flax seeds on your salads and veggies or add to your protein smoothies.

**Almonds and walnuts.** Nuts are loaded with fiber and contain unsaturated fat, both of which are beneficial to increase insulin sensitivity. Just one handful of almonds or walnuts will provide a feeling of satiety. Walnuts have two times the amount of antioxidants compared to other nuts, and have two to fifteen times more potency than vitamin E in terms of antioxidant capacity. They contain high levels of glutathione (a potent antioxidant), L-arginine (an amino acid) and omega-3 fatty acids. Walnuts are an easy-to-pack-and-carry snack that will stabilize blood sugar and ward off hunger.

Beware that nuts can be problematic for some people, specifically those with autoimmune issues, allergies and digestive dysfunction. When purchasing nuts, opt for the raw version to avoid pesticide and mold exposure, and buy them in smaller quantities instead of the larger bins. Store nuts in the refrigerator in a glass jar and use them in a timely manner.

**Vegetables and leafy greens** are jam-packed with vitamins and minerals, phytonutrients (plant nutrients), chlorophyll, antioxidants, enzymes and soluble fiber.

The fiber found in vegetables and leafy greens contribute to post-meal feelings of satisfaction and fullness so you naturally eat less. A fiber-rich diet will maintain digestive health; support regularity, elimination and detoxification; excrete xenoestrogens from the body; reduce insulin and glucose levels; regulate weight and provide a sense of fullness.

Consuming leafy greens and vegetables encourages a healthy body composition, increases energy, boosts immunity, beautifies skin, prevents heart disease, fights cancer and accelerates fat loss.

Locally grown, organic veggies that are in-season are best. Avoid iceberg lettuce – not only is it void of nutrients, iceberg lettuce is often high in parasites.

A simple, delicious way to boost your fiber and veggie intake is with a nutrient-rich green smoothie. Juice or blend your favorite greens in a Vitamix or high-powered blender. Be sure to add a teaspoon of coconut oil, chia seeds or other healthy fat to ensure you absorb the nutrients from the greens.

**Fruits.** A study published in the *International Journal of Obesity* found that those who increased their intake of vegetables and low sugar fruits (berries, apples, nectarines, grapefruits) had a 24 percent lower risk of obesity.

**Berries** are a nutrient-rich superfood low in fructose and high in antioxidants, phytochemicals, polyphenols and fiber, that improve cognitive function and memory and promote fat loss. The polyphenols in blueberries inhibit the formation of new fats cells and help in the process to break down stored fat.

**Avocados** are a fruit jam-packed with healthy monounsaturated fat, antioxidants, phytonutrients, minerals, enzymes and fiber. Avocados are also a good source of energy-producing vitamin B5 and muscle-healthy potassium; in fact, they are higher in potassium than a medium banana. An excellent anti-inflammatory fruit, avocados are rich in glutathione-producing compounds that actively promote liver health by protecting the liver against toxic overload.

Research has found that adding avocado or avocado oil to a salad or other nutritious meals increases nutrient absorption. It's important to remember that it is not just the presence of nutrients in foods that matter, it is also the body's ability to absorb these nutrients. Adding half an avocado to a salad of romaine lettuce, spinach and carrots increases absorption of carotenoids from this salad between 200-400 percent. Interestingly, adding avocado to salsa increased carotenoid absorption from the salsa as well.

Next time you make a salad, add some avocado and you'll absorb five times the nutrients of the other vegetables.

**Lemons and limes** are rich in vitamins, minerals and antioxidants. They are nourishing for your liver, cleanse the body of unhealthy toxins, aid in digestion, promote alkalinity, and can reduce blood sugar levels by as much as thirty percent. Before meals, drink a cup of water with the juice of a fresh lemon or lime to promote healthy digestion. Or, squeeze fresh lemon or lime on your salad or fish.

**Grapefruit** contains phytochemicals that help reduce insulin levels and increase the flow of digestive juices in the stomach. Grapefruits are rich in vitamin C and antioxidants. They contain a flavonoid compound called naringenin that causes the liver to burn fat rather than store it. Eaten at the beginning of a meal, grapefruit aids in digestion and can help with fat loss.

## Beverages for a Hot 'n Healthy Body

**Water** is one of the most important nutrients and often overlooked for detoxification, losing body fat and optimal health. Your body is approximately 70% water, brain tissue is 75% water, and blood is 83% water.

Water is an ally for fat loss that is calorie-free, naturally suppresses appetite and aids in detoxification and fat metabolism. Drinking cold water can increase your metabolism temporarily. Dehydration raises cortisol, which can signal the body to store body fat around the mid-section. In a study, those who drank two cups of water before each meal lost an average of five pounds more weight over a 12-week calorie-controlled diet than those who followed the same diet but did not drink the water.

Without sufficient water intake, your kidneys are unable to function properly, which forces them to send some of the workload to your liver.

Since one of main functions of the liver is to metabolize stored fat, the added workload passed on from the kidneys means that the liver metabolizes less fat. As a result, more fat is stored.

Non-filtered water contains toxic chemicals, including chlorine and fluoride, which is a cumulative poison that causes many common health problems including dementia, reduced IQ, increased lead absorption, hypothyroid, bone, brain and thyroid cancer, bone fractures, depression and obesity.

Aim for a minimum of half your body weight in ounces of filtered water every day, even more if you're athletic or live in a hot climate. To determine the number of ounces you should be drinking every day, take your body weight and multiply by .7. This formula provides you with your personal daily water requirements.

Enhance the flavor of water by adding any of the following alone or in combination: raspberries, ginger, cucumbers, lemons, limes or fresh mint. You can also add a pinch of unprocessed sea salt for additional minerals.

**Green tea.** Catechins, particularly EGCG, a potent antioxidant found in green tea, contain anti-inflammatory, anti-cancer and fat oxidation benefits. Green tea can help speed recovery from exercise because the antioxidants found in green tea reduce inflammation and neutralize free radical oxidation that occurs with intense exercising.

A study published in the *Journal of Clinical Nutrition* proved that high daily amounts of the fat burning catechins found in green tea stimulate metabolism and accelerate fat loss. The results of the study suggest that consumption of a beverage containing green tea catechins enhances weight loss, reduces triglycerides and decreases abdominal fat as compared to those on a control beverage without the green tea catechins.

Six cups of fresh-brewed, non-fluoridated, organic green tea daily (or take standardized green tea extract supplements) will help you lose weight and increase your fat loss efforts.

Be sure the tea is organic as a number of tea brands are laced with toxic pesticides. Many brands of tea are also high in fluoride, which can displace iodine in the thyroid gland, exacerbating hypothyroidism and the inability to lose weight. Regardless of whether the tea is organic or not, the fluoride content is linked to the soil in which the tea was grown.

**Coffee** contains a blend of free-radical fighting antioxidants, bioflavonoids, vitamins and minerals. Moderate consumption of organic, pesticide-free coffee can increase insulin sensitivity and metabolic rate and reduce risk of diabetes and Parkinson's disease. A study published in the *Molecular Nutrition & Food Research* journal showed that those who drank four cups of coffee daily lost 1.5 pounds of body fat in four weeks.

Enjoy your coffee prior to your workout, NOT after, to boost performance, increase energy and mobilize fat stores. Consuming coffee after your workout increases cortisol and interferes with your body's ability to recover and build muscle.

We are all different and people metabolize caffeine differently. While consuming coffee can be beneficial for some, you can drink too much of a good thing. Coffee should be avoided by women with fibrocystic breast disease and are pregnant or breastfeeding, and anyone at risk of osteoporosis, taking prescription medications, or suffering from adrenal fatigue.

## On the side

**Apple cider vinegar** has been highly regarded throughout history. In 400 B.C., the great Hippocrates, Father of Medicine, used it for its amazing health qualities. Apple cider vinegar contains acetic acid, which slows the passage of food from the stomach into the small intestine. Acetic acid is associated with numerous health benefits including increased HDL, lower LDL and reduced liver fats, and aids in less fat accumulation.

A small amount of apple cider vinegar in water before meals supports digestion and pH balance, improves satiety and prevents overeating by suppressing appetite. Apple cider vinegar also lowers the glycemic load of a meal, improves insulin sensitivity and prevents fluctuations in blood sugar that can influence weight loss, especially for diabetics and those who are insulin resistant.

A 2009 study published in the *Journal of Agriculture Food and Chemistry* found that subjects who consumed acetic acid for 12 weeks experienced significant declines in body weight, abdominal fat, waist circumference and triglycerides. When purchasing apple cider vinegar, opt for organic, unfiltered, unheated, unpasteurized apple cider vinegar.

**Cocoa and cacao** contain rich sources of flavonoids, antioxidants and magnesium. Flavanoids support cellular and metabolic functions throughout the body by providing antioxidant support and reducing inflammation. A study published in the *Journal of Nutrition* concluded that flavanoid-rich cocoa consumption has a positive influence on cholesterol, blood pressure and insulin resistance.

According to this study, cocoa flavanols may also help improve the appearance of women's skin by increasing hydration, decreasing skin roughness and protecting against UV damage.

Cacao is a natural anti-depressant that encourages the release of serotonin and stimulates secretion of endorphins that aid in relieving stress. Dark chocolate with a cocoa content of at least 70 percent is a tasty treat that reduces oxidative stress, lowers inflammation, boosts memory and cognitive function and helps eliminate cravings.

**Cinnamon** is a great tasting, powerful spice with numerous health benefits. Cinnamon helps control post-meal insulin spikes, reducing the glycemic index of a meal up to 29 percent. Cinnamon supports digestion, stabilized blood sugar, boosts metabolism and increases insulin sensitivity. Sprinkle cinnamon in coffee, smoothies, or post-workout shake, or enjoy a cup of cinnamon tea.

**Turn up the heat.** Chili peppers, jalapeños, cayenne, and hot, spicy mustard contain capsaicin, the substance that makes chili peppers spicy. There is a positive correlation between ingesting capsaicin and accelerated metabolic rate and fat loss.

Capsaicin causes thermogenesis (fat burning), which is responsible for amping up your metabolism and decreasing appetite and food intake. As a matter of fact, dietary consumption of capsaicin foods can increase metabolic rate by five to ten percent for up to two hours after eating them, and increase fat burning up to 16 percent.

Aside from capsaicin, other thermogenic foods include:
*   Protein
*   Turmeric (curcumin)
*   Caffeinated coffee
*   Various teas, including Yerba mate, green, white and oolong

## What's on the menu?

The *Fat Loss Revolution* menu plan will stabilize blood sugar, reduce cravings, increase energy, provide fuel for your brain, satisfy taste buds, balance your hormones, improve body composition and accelerate fat loss.

The menu options for breakfast, lunch, dinner and snacks follow the PVFC method, and are balanced, nutrient-rich meals that include a healthy combination of protein; fibrous, non-starchy carbohydrates; and healthy fats.

Choose to eat the majority of your meals at home versus eating out at a restaurant as often as possible. Preparing and cooking your meals at home ensures that you are eating higher quality foods, you're aware of the ingredients used and you can use healthier cooking methods.

## Breakfast
Starting with breakfast, I cannot fail to mention coffee. By all means enjoy your morning cup of coffee.

### For the love of coffee
If you enjoy having your java, here are a few key points to keep in mind:
* Refrain from drinking coffee on an empty stomach first thing in the morning.
* Eat breakfast before your morning cup of java.
* Coffee should be organic.
* Rotate brands of coffee. When you finish one specific brand, switch to a different brand.
* Use a small amount of organic, heavy whipping cream or coconut creamer if you opt for a creamer
* Avoid all non-fat, low-fat and flavored creamers.
* Need to sweeten your coffee? Opt for stevia powder or liquid plain or flavored stevia such as *Sweet Leaf Stevia.*

# Breakfast options for a Hot 'n Healthy Body

See *Chapter 15* for recipes.

Reminders:

* The size of a deck of cards is equivalent to approximately 20-25 grams of protein. One egg contains six grams of protein.

* Females – aim for 40-50 grams of protein before lunch.

* Males – aim for 50-70 grams of protein before lunch.

Before you eat breakfast:

* Mix three tablespoons of soluble fiber powder and a sprinkle of cinnamon with six ounces of water and drink quickly. Drink six to eight more ounces of water.

* Drink one cup (approximately six to eight ounces) of water with the juice of one-half fresh lemon or one whole lime

Choose one of the breakfast options below. Rotate these options daily.

_____ ◈ _____

Organic whole eggs with spinach and tomatoes
1/4 avocado
Blueberries

_____ ◈ _____

Coconut pancakes
Organic nitrate-free chicken apple sausage
Raspberries

_____ ◈ _____

Mean 'n Green Smoothie

_____ ◈ _____

---◈---

Apple nut salad
Bunless turkey or bison burger

---◈---

Turkey Apple Walnut Goodness

---◈---

Baked Florentine Egg Cups

---◈---

Organic, grass-fed animal protein (beef, bison, ostrich, elk)
Veggies, steamed or sautéed, such as asparagus, red bell pepper, onion
and garlic

---◈---

Full-fat Greek or coconut yogurt, add 1 scoop Whey Cool or Vital
whey protein powder, frozen berries, chia seeds and cinnamon

---◈---

Three organic whole eggs plus three additional whites
Sautéed kale, mushrooms and onions
Blackberries

---◈---

Grilled chicken breast
Spinach, steamed or sautéed
Handful of pecans

---◈---

*See page 51 for more breakfast ideas.*

## Lunch options for a hot 'n healthy body

See *Chapter 15* for recipes.

_____ ◈ _____

Chicken, Pecan and Pear Salad

_____ ◈ _____

Juicy, grass-fed bison or beef burger with large, dark green salad

_____ ◈ _____

Kale Salad with Wild Salmon

_____ ◈ _____

In a large collard green, wrap up sliced chicken breast, pomegranate seeds, broccoli sprouts, cucumber slices, avocado and chia seeds

_____ ◈ _____

Chopped chicken breast, salsa and avocado wrapped in bibb lettuce

_____ ◈ _____

Large chicken breast placed atop a dark, green leafy salad such as arugula or spinach with olive oil and apple cider vinegar or balsamic vinegar dressing

_____ ◈ _____

Eight large shrimp sautéed in coconut oil and garlic and sprinkled with fresh parmesan cheese. Place atop your favorite dark, leafy green salad such as kale with freshly chopped basil and freshly chopped mint. Drizzle with olive oil and the juice from a freshly squeezed lime or lemon.

_____ ◈ _____

## Dinner options for a hot 'n healthy body

See *Chapter 15* for recipes.

———————————————— ◈ ————————————————

Wild Salmon with Asparagus and Mushrooms
———————————————— ◈ ————————————————

Tropical Shrimp Roll Up
———————————————— ◈ ————————————————

Turkey Spinach Meatloaf
Cauliflower Faux Potatoes
Green Beans Almondine
———————————————— ◈ ————————————————

Thai-style Chicken and Veggies with Quinoa
———————————————— ◈ ————————————————

Large chicken breast baked with rosemary, salt and pepper
Small yam or sweet potato with pastured butter
Broccoli, steamed, add olive oil and garlic
———————————————— ◈ ————————————————

Grilled halibut with lemon and freshly grated ginger
Roasted asparagus
Mixed green salad with lemon and olive oil
———————————————— ◈ ————————————————

Coconut Macadamia Chicken or Shrimp
Large, dark green salad with chopped purple cabbage and a chopped
Granny Smith apple with olive oil and rice wine vinegar
———————————————— ◈ ————————————————

## 25 surprisingly simple snacks for a hot 'n healthy body

1. Turkey with hot mustard wrapped around 2 stalks of steamed asparagus or baby broccoli

2. Almonds and macadamia nuts with crystallized ginger

3. Chocolate Raspberry Cocoa Smoothie (*see Chapter 15 for recipe*)

4. 1/2 of an avocado with fresh squeezed lemon juice

5. Organic chicken breast (chopped) and sliced avocado, rolled up in a chard or collard green leaf, with a potent cup of green tea

6. Cocoa Covered Walnuts (walnuts dusted with dark cocoa)

7. 2 scoops Chocolate Vital Whey protein powder, 1/2 cup coconut cream, 1 tsp. organic cocoa, 1 packet of Stevia Plus, 1 cup organic brewed coffee, and ice. Blend in Vitamix or high-powered blender.

8. Olive oil-based cilantro jalapeno hummus with sliced red bell peppers and cucumbers

9. Chopped green apples with walnuts, cinnamon and splash of apple cider vinegar

10. Green apple with macadamia nut butter sprinkled with cinnamon

11. Gluten-free Mary's Gone Crackers with almond butter (stir chia seeds into almond butter for added fiber and omega-3 fats)

12. Small piece of 70 percent dark chocolate with 1/2 cup organic raspberries

13. Handful of raw, organic almonds, walnuts or hazelnuts

14. 2 scoops Vital Whey vanilla protein powder, one scoop Greens First powder, one cup unsweetened almond or coconut milk, one cup filtered water and ice. Blend in blender or Vitamix.

15. Raw milk cheese with pears and pecans

16. Hardboiled eggs

17. Celery with raw cashew butter or almond butter

18. Brown rice tortilla drizzled with coconut oil, sprinkle of cinnamon, walnuts and chopped apple. Broil under broiler.

19. Potent cup of tea (green or Yerba Mate Royale tea) poured over ice

20. Sliced grapefruit and avocado

21. 1 cup blueberries with handful of cashews or pecans

22. Small bison burger (no bun) with sliced avocado and pico de gallo sauce or fresh salsa

23. Homemade kale chips (see *Chapter 15* for recipe)

24. 1 cup full-fat Greek or coconut yogurt, 1 scoop of vanilla Whey Cool or Vital Whey protein powder, 1/4 cup frozen raspberries, 1 tbsp. chia seeds

25. Organic turkey, chicken, beef, buffalo, bison or wild-caught salmon jerky

*Be proactive and prepare some healthy snacks and meals on the weekend so you have food readily available when you're busy throughout the week.*

# CHAPTER 14

## SHOPPING SOLUTIONS FOR A HOT 'N HEALTHY BODY

### 7 Solutions at the Supermarket

Here are seven solutions to make your supermarket shopping a healthier and easier experience.

**1. Become an avid label reader and read the list of ingredients on each and every product.** This is the most significant detail to pay attention to, but is often in small print.

Clever marketing and advertising distract most individuals to bypass reading the list of ingredients. The product manufacturer and marketers highlight what they want you to notice to entice you to buy their product. Products labeled organic, sugar-free, gluten-free, low-fat, or cholesterol-free can be deceptive and misleading. Items labeled as low-fat can trick you into thinking you're eating less. A box of sugary cereal may say "made from 100 percent whole grains" or "excellent source of fiber" or "gluten-free." This does not automatically give the green light that this product is a healthy one.

Most boxed cereals and many supermarket products contain processed grains, sugar, artificial sweeteners, chemical-laden dyes, preservatives, soy, genetically engineered ingredients, synthetic vitamins and other toxic substances.

Supermarket shelves are stocked primarily with processed and packaged foods. At least 90 percent of them contain an assortment of sugar, chemicals, soy, vegetable oils, wheat or GMOs. Foods that are refined and processed have been taken out of their natural context, destroying vitamins, minerals and important nutrients.

An informed label reader knows what to look for and which ingredients to avoid, such as high-fructose corn syrup, hydrolyzed yeast extract, aspartame, sucralose, enriched wheat flour, soybean oil, canola oil and partially-hydrogenated vegetable oils. Beware of gluten hiding in items such as soy sauce, mustard, ketchup, luncheon meats, soups, pickles and many other products.

Consider the following ingredients found on a box of crackers, which may seem healthy to you – with the translation of what the ingredients actually are in parentheses:

* Whole grain oats (sugar)
* Sugar (sugar)
* Vegetable oil (genetically-modified frankenfat)
* Rice flour (sugar)
* High maltose corn syrup (sugar)
* Honey (sugar)
* Rice maltodextrin (sugar)
* Salt (sodium chloride)
* Soy lecithin (an emulsifier and a byproduct of soybean oil)
* Milk (pasteurized, non-organic milk)
* Baking soda (baking soda)
* Barley malt extract (sugar)
* Natural flavoring (this can be anything)

As you can see, this product is not all that healthy after all. The take-away message is this: If you do not know what the ingredient is, or you cannot pronounce it, *do not buy the product!*

Most processed foods have natural and/or artificial flavors added to them during the production process. Flavors are made by flavorists in a laboratory, either by blending natural or synthetic chemicals together to enhance taste. Blending chemicals derived from a natural source, such as a plant or animal product, produces natural flavors. Combining synthetic (human-made) chemicals produces artificial flavors.

Therefore, the primary difference between natural and artificial flavorings is in the origin of the chemicals used to produce their tastes.

**2. Navigate the outer perimeter aisles of the supermarket** and stock up on plenty of staples, including grass-fed meats; organic, free-range poultry; wild fish and seafood; a wide array of organic, non-starchy vegetables and leafy greens; a variety of berries and low-gycemic fruits, teas, raw nuts, seeds, spices and herbs; full-fat yogurt; cocoa; coconut milk; olive oil and coconut oil.

**3. Shop at your local farmer's market, co-ops and farms,** where you'll find organic vegetables and fruits, and animal products with a higher nutritional value than those found in big supermarkets.

**4. Buy brightly colored vegetables and fruits** that are in season. Aim for a new fruit or vegetable every week.

**5. Eat a meal or protein-rich snack before you go shopping.** Do not go grocery shopping when you're hungry (low blood sugar).

**6. Shop with a shopping list.** Buy a variety of foods (see *Chapter 14*).

**7. Shop alone.** Research suggests that adults are more likely to buy high-calorie foods when they shop with their kids. You'll stick to your shopping list if you are on your own.

> *Do not buy any product that contains enriched wheat flour, soy bean oil, canola oil, partially-hydrogenated oils, high fructose corn syrup, autolyzed or hydrolyzed yeast extracts, aspartame, dextrose or anything ending in –ose, or any ingredient with a number next to it. Avoid low-fat and non-fat items.*

## Ingredients to avoid

Take this list with you when you go to the supermarket. Also, refer to *Chapter 7.*

☐ Acesulfame-K (acesulfame potassium)
☐ Ammonium chloride
☐ Any item on the label that is autolyzed or hydrolyzed
☐ Artificial colors (any color with a # sign)
☐ Artificial sweeteners including aspartame and saccharin
☐ Azodicarbonamide
☐ Benzoates, sodium benzoate
☐ BHA and BHT (butylated hydroxyanisole and butylated hydroxytoluene)
☐ Brominated vegetable oil
☐ Calcium saccharin and calcium stearoyl-2-lactylate
☐ Canola oil and other vegetable oils
☐ Cyclamates
☐ Dimethylpolysiloxane
☐ Ethoxyquin
☐ Ethylene oxide
☐ High-fructose corn syrup and corn syrup
☐ Hydrogenated oil and partially hydrogenated oil
☐ Maltodextrin
☐ Methyl silicon
☐ Monosodium glutamate (MSG)
☐ Polydextrose
☐ Potassium benzoate
☐ Propylparaben
☐ Silicon/titanium dioxide
☐ Soybean oil and soy
☐ Sulfites (sulfur dioxide) and sodium sulfite
☐ TBHQ (tertiary butylhydroquinone)
☐ Tetrasodium EDTA

# Your Hot 'n Healthy Shopping List

This list of healthy food options can be used as your supermarket shopping list. Shop for nutrient-dense whole foods; avoid foods that are processed and refined.

Make copies and check off the items you need to purchase.

## Protein – meat, eggs and seafood
Organic, free-range, pastured and grass-fed sources
☐ Applegate cold cuts (free of MSG)
☐ Beef
☐ Buffalo/bison
☐ Chicken
☐ Cornish hen
☐ Eggs
☐ Fish: Halibut, snapper, trout, wild salmon, catfish, sardines
☐ Other seafood
☐ Lobster, shrimp, crab, prawns
☐ Lamb
☐ Bacon and turkey bacon
☐ Chicken and turkey sausage, nitrate-free
☐ Ostrich
☐ Turkey
☐ Venison
☐ Whey protein (please visit PaulaOwens.com)

## Vegetables and leafy greens

Any item *italicized* indicates to buy as organic only according to the EWG's Dirty Dozen list (*see page 104*).

### Vegetables

- [ ] Alfalfa sprouts
- [ ] Artichokes
- [ ] Asparagus
- [ ] Bamboo shoots
- [ ] Beets
- [ ] *Bell peppers*
- [ ] Bok choy
- [ ] Broccoli
- [ ] Brussel sprouts
- [ ] Cabbage
- [ ] Carrot
- [ ] Cauliflower
- [ ] *Celery*
- [ ] Chives
- [ ] Cucumber
- [ ] Eggplant
- [ ] Green beans
- [ ] Jicama
- [ ] Leeks
- [ ] Mushrooms
- [ ] Onions
- [ ] Radish
- [ ] Seaweed
- [ ] Snap peas
- [ ] Squash (green, yellow)
- [ ] Spaghetti squash
- [ ] String beans
- [ ] Tomato
- [ ] Turnips
- [ ] Water chestnuts
- [ ] Zucchini

### Leafy greens

- [ ] Arugula
- [ ] Beet greens
- [ ] Chard
- [ ] Cilantro
- [ ] *Collard greens*
- [ ] Dandelion
- [ ] Endive
- [ ] Escarole
- [ ] *Kale*
- [ ] Mustard greens
- [ ] Parsley
- [ ] Purslane
- [ ] Radicchio
- [ ] *Red or green loose-leaf lettuce*
- [ ] *Romaine lettuce*
- [ ] *Spinach*
- [ ] Turnip greens
- [ ] Watercress

## Fruits

- ☐ *Apples*
- ☐ Apricot
- ☐ Avocado
- ☐ Banana
- ☐ *Blackberries*
- ☐ *Blueberries*
- ☐ Coconut
- ☐ Cranberries
- ☐ Dark cherries
- ☐ Figs
- ☐ Grapefruit
- ☐ *Grapes*
- ☐ Guava
- ☐ Kiwi
- ☐ Lemon
- ☐ Lime
- ☐ Mango
- ☐ *Nectarine*
- ☐ Oranges
- ☐ Papaya
- ☐ *Peaches*
- ☐ Pears
- ☐ Pineapple
- ☐ Plums
- ☐ Pomegranate
- ☐ *Raspberries*
- ☐ *Strawberries*
- ☐ Tangerine
- ☐ Watermelon

## Grains, legumes and potatoes

(if not intolerant to lectins)

- ☐ Black beans, pinto, legumes, lentils or other beans
- ☐ Oatmeal, gluten-free
- ☐ Quinoa (which is actually a seed), amaranth, teff
- ☐ *Red, organic potato*
- ☐ Rice (brown, white, black or red)
- ☐ *Sweet potato*
- ☐ Yam

## Beverages

- ☐ Almond milk (unsweetened)
- ☐ Coconut creamer
- ☐ Coconut milk
- ☐ Coconut water
- ☐ *Coffee, organic*
- ☐ Hemp milk
- ☐ Seltzer water with flavored Stevia
- ☐ Water
- ☐ Herbal teas
- ☐ Pau 'd Arco tea
- ☐ Dandelion
- ☐ Peppermint
- ☐ *Green tea*
- ☐ *White tea*
- ☐ Yerba Mate tea

## Herbs and spices

- [ ] Basil
- [ ] Bay leaf
- [ ] Caraway
- [ ] Cardamom
- [ ] Cayenne
- [ ] Chili pepper
- [ ] Chipolte
- [ ] Chives
- [ ] Cilantro
- [ ] Cinnamon
- [ ] Clove
- [ ] Coriander
- [ ] Cumin
- [ ] Curry
- [ ] Dill
- [ ] Fennel
- [ ] Fenugreek
- [ ] Garlic
- [ ] Ginger
- [ ] Lemongrass
- [ ] Licorice
- [ ] Marjoram
- [ ] Mint
- [ ] Mustard
- [ ] Oregano
- [ ] Sea salt, unprocessed
- [ ] Paprika
- [ ] Parsley
- [ ] Pepper, Black
- [ ] Peppermint
- [ ] Rosemary
- [ ] Saffron
- [ ] Spearmint
- [ ] Tarragon
- [ ] Thyme
- [ ] Turmeric
- [ ] Vanilla
- [ ] Wasabi

## Fats and oils

- [ ] Avocado oil
- [ ] Butter
- [ ] Ghee
- [ ] Virgin coconut oil
- [ ] Macadamia nut oil
- [ ] Extra-virgin olive oil
- [ ] Red palm oil
- [ ] Walnut oil

## Nuts, seeds and nut butters

(organic, raw)

- [ ] Almond
- [ ] Brazil nut
- [ ] Chia
- [ ] Flax
- [ ] Hazelnut
- [ ] Macadamia
- [ ] Pecan
- [ ] Pine
- [ ] Pistachio
- [ ] Pumpkin
- [ ] Sunflower
- [ ] Walnut

## Condiments and miscellaneous

- ☐ Almond flour
- ☐ Apple cider vinegar
- ☐ Cacao (cocoa)
- ☐ Chocolate (dark)
  (minimum 70% cacao)
- ☐ Cocoa nibs
- ☐ Coconut flakes
- ☐ Coconut flour
- ☐ Coconut sugar
- ☐ Coconut yogurt
- ☐ *Greek yogurt (full fat)*
- ☐ Honey
- ☐ Horseradish
- ☐ Hummus (olive oil-based)
- ☐ Kefir
- ☐ Kombucha
- ☐ Maple syrup
- ☐ Mary's Gone Crackers
- ☐ Mustard
- ☐ Salsa
- ☐ Stevia Plus or liquid Stevia
- ☐ Tabasco
- ☐ Vegetable and chicken broth
  (low sodium)

## Other items

- ☐ _____
- ☐ _____
- ☐ _____
- ☐ _____
- ☐ _____
- ☐ _____
- ☐ _____
- ☐ _____
- ☐ _____
- ☐ _____

# CHAPTER 15

## DELICIOUS RECIPES FOR A HOT 'N HEALTHY BODY

* Coconut Pancakes (p. 310)
* Baked Florentine Egg Cups (p. 311)
* Get Lean Green Smoothie (p. 311)
* Mean 'n Green Fat Loss Smoothie (p. 312)
* Turkey Apple Walnut Goodness (p. 313)
* Kale Chips (p. 313)
* Cilantro-Lime Dressing (p. 314)
* Nutty Besto Pesto (p. 315)
* Oh-So-Yummy Granola (p. 316)
* Chocolate Raspberry Cocoa Smoothie (p. 317)
* Nutty Apple Salad (p. 317)
* Quick and Tasty Spinach (p. 318)
* Roasted Asparagus (p. 318)
* Green Bean Almondine (p. 319)
* Cauliflower Faux-tatoes (p. 319)
* Coconut Macadamia Chicken or Shrimp (p. 320)
* Tropical Shrimp Rollup (p. 321)
* Chicken, Pecan and Pear Salad (p. 322)
* Kale Salad with Wild Salmon (p. 323)
* Broiled Salmon with Asparagus and Mushrooms (p. 324)
* Braised Bacon Apple Cabbage (p. 325)
* Juicy Grass-fed Beef or Bison Burgers (p. 326)
* Thai-style Chicken and Veggies with Quinoa (p. 327)
* Bison, Beef or Turkey and Spinach Meatloaf (p. 328)
* Strawberry Ice Cream with Dark Chocolate (p. 328)

## Coconut Pancakes

Enjoy these pancakes with your favorite berries or wrap up some bacon and eggs or your favorite chicken sausage for a healthier breakfast burrito. Or just eat them plain.

4 whole organic eggs
1/4 cup coconut flour
1/4 tsp. vanilla extract
1 pinch nutmeg
1 tsp. cinnamon
1 tbsp. raw honey
1/4 cup coconut milk

Mix the ingredients and let it sit for 5 minutes. Add a small amount of coconut oil or butter to your pan and heat over medium heat. Pour about a 1/4 cup of batter for each pancake. Allow to brown before flipping.

♥_____♥

## Baked Florentine Egg Cups

    12 fresh organic eggs
    12 thin slices of turkey
    1 cup fresh spinach
    1/2 cup scallions, diced
    Sea salt and pepper
    Coconut oil

Preheat oven to 400°. Lightly wipe each muffin tin hole with a thin layer of coconut oil. Place a piece of turkey into each hole creating a little cup. Place some of the fresh spinach in each turkey cup. Crack 1 egg into each hole and top with a couple of diced scallions. Sprinkle with salt and pepper. Bake for 12 minutes until white is firm.

♥_____♥

## Get Lean Green Smoothie

In a Vitamix or high-powered blender, add the following ingredients:

    1 cup water or coconut water
    2" piece of fresh ginger root
    1/4 cucumber, sliced
    1 carrot, sliced
    1/2 green apple
    Fresh parsley
    5-6 leaves kale

After the veggies are blended and liquefied, add the following:

    Ice
    30 grams protein powder
    2 tsp. coconut oil

Blend until ice is liquefied.

♥_____♥

## Mean 'n Green Fat Loss Smoothie

In a Vitamix or high-powered blender, add the following ingredients:

1 cup water or coconut water
1/4 cup aloe vera juice
1 celery stalk
Fresh ginger root
3-4 kale leaves
1/2 green apple
1/4 cucumber
4 dandelion stalks (awesome for the liver)
Handful fresh Italian parsley
Watercress (excellent for detoxing estrogens)
Fresh cilantro (great for chelating heavy metals)
Juice from a whole lime

After the veggies are blended and liquefied, add the following:

Ice
30 grams protein powder
2 tsp. coconut oil

Blend until ice is liquefied.

Other leafy greens and veggies I like blending include Swiss chard, spinach, asparagus, carrots and beets. I seldom use fruit and focus more on veggies and leafy greens.

♥_____♥

## Turkey Apple Walnut Goodness

Courtesy of Evelyne Lambrecht, Health Coach, San Diego

1/2 to 1 apple, chopped into bite-size chunks
4-6 ounces nitrate-free chicken or turkey sausage
1/4 cup walnuts
Coconut oil
Cinnamon

Melt some organic, unsalted butter, ghee or coconut oil in a pan. Add the apple and allow to sauté for a while, then add the sausage. Stir it all together. Sauté until the apple pieces begin to brown and start getting just a bit soft. Last, add the walnuts and let everything heat up for a little longer. Serve with some black pepper or sprinkle with cinnamon.

This is a great breakfast dish because it keeps you full for a while and has a good amount of protein, fat and fiber to keep your blood sugar stable. Plus, it's gluten-free!

♥_____♥


## Kale Chips

1 lb. kale, chopped
Olive oil

Preheat oven to 200°. Place kale in large bowl. Add 3 tbsp. olive oil and toss to coat kale leaves. Line a baking sheet with parchment paper. Spread kale onto baking sheet. Roast for approximately 30-35 minutes until crisp. Turn leaves every 10 minutes.

Optional: When done, sprinkle unprocessed sea salt, garlic, balsamic vinegar or your other favorite spice or herb into the bowl of kale.

♥_____♥

## Cilantro-Lime Dressing

2 tbsp. extra virgin olive oil
1 tbsp. onion, minced
1 tbsp. cilantro, chopped
3 tbsp. fresh lime juice (about the juice of one lime)
1 tsp. Dijon mustard
1/4 tsp. sea salt
1/4 tsp. black pepper
1 garlic clove, crushed or minced

Blend ingredients in Vitamix or blender for 1 to 2 minutes until smooth.

Enjoy this salad dressing on your favorite leafy green salad. Add:

Grilled chicken breast, shrimp or wild salmon
Walnuts or pecans
Red onion, sliced
Avocado, chopped

♥_____♥

## Nutty Besto Pesto

3-4 cloves garlic (may use frozen crushed garlic cubes)
1/3 cup Brazil nuts
1/3 cup macadamia nuts
1/3 cup walnuts
1/3 cup sunflower seeds
1/3 cup pumpkin seeds
1 cup fresh basil
1 cup fresh cilantro
1 cup parsley
3/4 - 1 cup cold pressed olive oil
Fresh lemon juice from the juice of an entire lemon
Pinch of sea salt

Soak the nuts and seeds overnight (doing so releases the enzyme exhibitors). In a food processor or Vitamix, combine the basil, cilantro, parsley and olive oil. Blend until smooth. Add the garlic, nuts, seeds, salt and lemon juice. Mix until the ingredients form a paste. Store the pesto in a glass container. Enjoy with your favorite veggie, seafood, poultry or with eggs. A little goes a long way.

Bonus: Nutty Besto Pesto is a natural heavy metal chelator, helpful for detoxing heavy metals from the body.

♥_____♥

## Oh-So-Yummy Granola

This quick and easy granola recipe is tasty, full of fiber and healthy. Great as a dessert and a treat kids love.

Preheat oven to 350°. Mix the following ingredients together and spread onto cookie sheet:

    2 cups old-fashioned, whole, organic, gluten-free oats
    1 heaping cup organic whole nuts (almonds, pecans)
    1/2 cup pumpkin seeds
    1 cup unsweetened flaked coconut
    2 tsp. cinnamon

Drizzle the following items over the above mixture:
    6 tbsp. organic maple syrup
    1 tsp. vanilla extract
    6 tbsp. coconut oil

Bake 25-30 minutes. Make sure to stir the granola every 5 minutes while cooking. When granola is golden, remove from oven.

Optional: Stir in 1 cup of your favorite sulfite-free dried fruit, such as chopped papaya or cherries.

Serve with organic, unsweetened coconut milk or by itself.

♥_____♥

## Chocolate Raspberry Cocoa Smoothie

In a Vitamix or high-powered blender, add the following ingredients:

2 scoops chocolate Vital Whey or Whey Cool protein powder
or Chocolate Mediclear SGS
1 cup chocolate coconut milk
1 cup filtered water
2/3 cup frozen organic raspberries
2 tbsp. raw, organic cacao nibs
Ice

Blend thoroughly and enjoy!

♥_____♥


## Nutty Apple Salad

Mix the following ingredients together in a bowl. Enjoy as a snack or for breakfast with your favorite protein source.

1 green apple, cored and chopped
1 red apple, cored and chopped
1/2 cup walnuts
1-1/2 cups full fat coconut yogurt
1 tbsp. chia seeds
a sprinkle of cinnamon

Optional: May add 1 cup of chicken breast, grilled and chopped.

♥_____♥

## Quick and Tasty Spinach

Courtesy of Maria DePasquale, Health Coach, Florida

1 bunch spinach
2-3 cloves garlic, minced
1 tbsp. organic, real butter

Rinse spinach thoroughly. Remove stems. In a large pan, sauté butter and garlic; add the spinach. Cook for a few minutes. Remove from heat and serve with your favorite protein source.

♥_____♥

## Roasted Asparagus

Courtesy of Maria DePasquale, Health Coach, Florida

2 cloves garlic minced
1/4 tsp. unprocessed Celtic sea salt
1 bunch asparagus, rinsed and fibrous ends cut off
1/8 tsp. red pepper flakes
1 tbsp. extra virgin olive oil
1-2 tsp. organic, raw parmesan cheese

Sprinkle sea salt, red pepper flakes and parmesan cheese on asparagus. Roast asparagus on grill or under broiler for 5 to 10 minutes. Let cool, then drizzle olive oil over asparagus and serve with your favorite protein.

♥_____♥

## Green Bean Almondine

Courtesy of Maria DePasquale, Health Coach, Florida

1 tbsp. real, organic butter
2 tbsp. slivered almonds
1 lb. fresh string beans, trimmed and blanched
2 shallots

Steam green beans in a steamer. When al dente, remove from steamer and immediately run under cold water. Place in a bowl and set aside. In a large pan, heat up the butter and shallots, and add your favorite spices. When the shallots appear translucent, add the slivered almonds until toasted. Add green beans and toss. Serve with your favorite protein.

♥_____♥

## Cauliflower Faux-tatoes

Courtesy of Maria DePasquale, Health Coach, Florida

1 large head cauliflower, boiled and mashed
2 strips bacon, chopped (optional)
1 bunch scallions, diced (optional)
1 tomato, diced (optional)
1 tsp. fresh garlic, chopped or one frozen garlic cube
1 tbsp. real, organic butter
2 tbsp. organic heavy cream

Steam the cauliflower until tender. Mash to consistency of mashed potatoes. Add the bacon, scallions, garlic, tomatoes and butter. Mix well. If you like this, it's a nice break from steamed vegetables.

Note: The nutrient water left over from steaming the cauliflower can be used instead of heavy cream.

♥_____♥

# Coconut Chicken or Shrimp Macadamia

- 1-2 cups unsweetened, organic, shredded coconut
- 1-2 cups raw, unsalted macadamia nuts, crushed
- 1 cup coconut milk
- Pinch unprocessed sea salt
- 1-1/2 to 2 lbs. organic chicken breast tenders or wild shrimp
- 1 tsp. organic coconut oil

Marinate chicken breast in coconut milk for 3 to 8 hours. Preheat oven to 350°. Coat a glass baking dish with coconut oil. Mix crushed macadamia nuts and shredded coconut in bowl. Roll chicken breast in coconut/macadamia mixture and place in baking dish.

Bake for 35-45 minutes (baking time varies according to different ovens). Serve with a dark green salad and asparagus or another veggie of your choice.

Optional: serve with quinoa.

♥_____♥

## Tropical Shrimp Roll Up

    1 lb. extra-large frozen cooked wild shrimp, cleaned and
        de-veined
    1 tsp. red pepper flakes
    2 mangoes, peeled, seeded and diced
    2 papayas, peeled, seeded and diced
    1/4 cup red onion, chopped
    1 small jalapeno pepper, seeded and finely chopped
    1 avocado, chopped
    1/2 cup cilantro, chopped
    2 large limes

Defrost shrimp under cold running water and pat dry. Place in bowl.
Squeeze juice from one of the limes over shrimp. Sprinkle red pepper
flakes over shrimp.

In a separate bowl, toss the mango, papaya, onion, jalapeno pepper,
avocado, cilantro and juice of 1 lime together.

Top your favorite green (Swiss chard, collard green, romaine or Bibb
lettuce leaves) with some of the shrimp and tropical mix. Roll it up
and enjoy!

♥_____♥

## Chicken Pecan-Pear Salad

2 organic pears, chopped and cored
3 cups watercress
3 cups arugula
1 cup fresh basil, chopped
1 cup fresh mint, chopped
1 cup fresh cilantro, chopped
1/2 cup pecans
1/2 cup red onion, chopped
1/4 cup gorgonzola cheese (optional)
1 – 2 lbs. organic chicken breast, grilled and chopped
1/2 cup olive oil
Juice from one whole lemon
Sea salt and pepper to taste

Place watercress, arugula, pecans, chicken, red onion and gorgonzola, salt, pepper, lemon and olive oil in large bowl. Toss until all of the ingredients are coated. Serve and enjoy.

♥_____♥

## Kale Salad with Wild Salmon

1 lb. kale, chopped
1/2 cup pine nuts
1 tomato, chopped
1/2 cup pomegranate seeds
1/4 cup chia seeds or freshly ground flax seed (optional)
1/2 cup olive oil
Juice from one whole lemon
Sea salt and pepper to taste
1 – 2 lbs. organic, wild salmon, grilled with your favorite
　　spices and lemon juice

Place kale, pine nuts, tomato, pomegranate seeds and chia seeds in large bowl. Sprinkle with salt and pepper. Pour olive oil and lemon over all and toss until coated.

Place some greens on your plate with a piece of the salmon on top.

♥_____♥

## Broiled Wild Salmon with Asparagus and Mushrooms
Courtesy of Cate Munroe, Cate's Nutrition Kitchen

1 lb. wild salmon filets
12 oz. asparagus, cut 2 inches off the bottom
6 oz. Portobello mushrooms, cut into 1 inch slices
2 tbsp. pastured butter
Sea salt and pepper to taste

Preheat broiler. Season both sides of salmon filets. Lay salmon skin-side up on a rimmed baking sheet (use foil for less clean up) 4 inches (or top rack) from the broiler. Broil for 4 to 5 minutes per side or until a fork can easily peel away flakes from the skin. Transfer to a large plate, top with 1 tbsp. butter, cover and let rest for 5 to 10 minutes.

While the salmon rests, spread asparagus and mushroom slices in a single layer on a rimmed baking sheet. Place 4 inches from the broiler. Broil for 4 to 5 minutes; flip vegetables to other side. Broil for 3 more minutes or until lightly golden brown and a fork can easily be inserted. Toss with butter, salt and pepper.

♥_____♥

## Braised Bacon Apple Cabbage

Courtesy of Cate Munroe, Cate's Nutrition Kitchen

4 slices pastured bacon
1 medium red onion, sliced thin
1 head green cabbage, sliced thin
1 tbsp. apple cider vinegar
1/2 cup water
1 Granny Smith apple, peeled, grated
Sea salt and pepper to taste

Heat a large stockpot or Dutch oven over medium heat for 5 minutes. Cook bacon until desired texture. Remove bacon, leaving as much grease behind as possible. Add onion and sauté for 5 minutes or until glossy. Add cabbage, vinegar and water. Cover and cook for 10 minutes or until the cabbage is tender. Stir in apple and chopped bacon. Season and serve hot or cold.

♥_____♥

## Juicy Grass-fed Beef or Bison Burgers

Courtesy of Cate Munroe, Cate's Nutrition Kitchen

2 lb. ground grass-fed beef or grass-fed bison
1 tbsp. coconut oil
1 tsp. each cayenne, garlic, ginger or chili, and cumin
1 tbsp. Tamari
4 scallions, minced

Preheat the broiler. Combine all ingredients in a large bowl. Form into 4 even-sized patties. Use your finger to create an indention in the middle of each burger (this ensures more even cooking). Broil for 8 minutes; flip and broil for 5 more minutes. Cover and let rest for 5 minutes before enjoying.

Serving suggestions:
Lettuce wrapped with tomato, pickled jalapeños, avocado and mustard
Raw milk cheese, caramelized onions and mushrooms
Wrapped with bacon, avocado and tomato
Broiled asparagus and red peppers
Chunky guacamole and tomato salsa

♥_____♥

# Thai-style Chicken and Veggies with Quinoa

1 lb. chicken breast tenders, grilled and chopped
1 cup cooked quinoa
1 cup steamed snow peas
1 cup steamed broccoli
1/2 cup coconut milk
1/4 cup natural, organic almond butter
1 tsp. sesame oil
1-2 tbsp. Tamari sauce
1-2 tbsp. fresh ground ginger
1 crushed clove of garlic
1/2 small avocado, diced into small pieces

Cook quinoa in 2 cups of water or chicken stock until the liquid has been absorbed, about 20 minutes. Set aside. Do not attempt to fluff the quinoa until it is cooled, as it can turn to mush easily when hot.

While the quinoa is cooking, begin steaming the snow peas and broccoli. Vegetables should be crisp-tender so they maintain the majority of their vitamins and minerals, as well as their fiber content. They should have a bright green color when finished steaming.

Sauce: Combine the coconut milk, almond butter, sesame oil, Tamari sauce, ginger and garlic in a small sauce pan. Over low heat, slowly stir with a wooden spoon until all are blended into a uniform sauce.

Mix the quinoa, veggies, chicken and Thai-style sauce in a large bowl or plate. Top with diced avocado.

♥_____♥

## Spinach Meatloaf

  1-1/2 lbs. turkey, beef or bison, ground
  2 eggs
  1 small onion, diced
  1-1/2 cups pecans, finely chopped
  2 cloves garlic or 2 frozen garlic cubes
  1/2 cup spinach, chopped and cooked
  1 tsp. dried basil or 2 tsp. fresh basil
  Sea salt and pepper to taste
  Coconut oil to coat baking dish

Preheat oven to 375. In large bowl, mix all of the ingredients. Place in
a glass baking dish that has been lightly coated with coconut oil.
Bake for 30 minutes. Remove from oven and allow to cool for 5
minutes before serving.

♥_____♥

## Strawberry Ice Cream with Dark Chocolate
Courtesy of Cate Munroe, Cate's Nutrition Kitchen

  1 cup organic heavy whipping cream or full-fat canned coconut
  milk
  Stevia (plain or flavored) to taste
  1 tsp. cinnamon
  2 tsp. vanilla, extract
  2 cups organic frozen strawberries
  1 frozen banana, peeled
  4 oz. dark chocolate (preferably 88%)

Combine all ingredients, except the chocolate and half of the fruit in a
blender. Blend for 1 minute, pushing down the edges with a spoon.
Add the remaining fruit. Blend for 2 more minutes or until thick and
creamy like soft-serve ice cream. Add more strawberries to thicken or
more cream or coconut milk to thin. Taste and adjust accordingly.
Enjoy with chocolate!

♥_____♥

# CHAPTER 16

# YOUR 12–WEEK CHECKLIST FOR A HOT 'N HEALTHY BODY

A written checklist can help you manage your *Fat Loss Revolution* and stay on track to reach your goals. Use this checklist in conjunction with the information in the *Fat Loss Revolution*.

Following is your weekly *Fat Loss Revolution* checklist for 12 weeks. Review your checklist every single day throughout the next 12 weeks.

## Before you start your 12-week *Fat Loss Revolution* plan

☐ Go through your kitchen and remove all of the processed foods and junk foods, such as white sugar, candy, pastries, white bread, soft drinks, pasteurized milk, vegetable oils, frozen dinners, non-organic meats, and any food or beverage containing wheat, soy, gluten, additives or artificial sweeteners. (pgs. 112-129)

☐ Plan your trip to the supermarket. Bring your hot 'n healthy shopping list (see *Chapter 14*).

☐ Take one day of the week to plan your weekly menu.

☐ Sign up at a local gym or get access to weight training equipment.

☐ Have your journals ready to record your food intake, measurements, workouts and daily gratitude list.

☐ Thoroughly read the checklist for week 1.

## Week 1

- ☐ Take your measurements and log them in your journal. (p. 13)
- ☐ Have your photos taken. (p. 14)
- ☐ Drink a cup of water with the juice of a lemon or lime before breakfast every morning.
- ☐ Eat breakfast. Include a quality protein source.
- ☐ Record all of your meals in your food journal.
- ☐ Lunch and dinner meals: follow the PFVC Method for your *Fat Loss Revolution* plate and make sure to include protein, a vegetable and/or dark leafy green salad. (p.150)
- ☐ Drink the appropriate number of ounces of clean, filtered water every day. (p. 288)
- ☐ Spend five minutes focusing on deep breathing.
- ☐ Get to bed no later than 10:00 p.m.
- ☐ Before bed, log in your gratitude journal.

◈ _____ ◈

## Week 2

- ☐ Continue with the checklist from week 1.
- ☐ Take your measurements and log them in your journal.
- ☐ Take updated photos.
- ☐ Start taking your primary essential supplements. (p. 275)
- ☐ Take the HCL test. (p. 96)
- ☐ Refrain from having temptation foods in your house.
- ☐ Practice some of the "Stress-less" strategies. (pgs. 73-79)
- ☐ If you have trouble sleeping, try any of the sleep tips found on pages 82-86.
- ☐ Take a 20-30 minute walk after dinner.
- ☐ Be proactive and prepare some healthy snacks and meals on the weekend so you have food readily available when you're busy during the week.

◈ _____ ◈

## Week 3

☐ Continue with the checklist from the prior weeks.

☐ Take your measurements and log them in your journal.

☐ Take updated photos.

☐ Minimize exposure to hidden obesogens in your diet and environment, including plastic bottles, sodas, soy, pesticides, non-organic meats, etc.

☐ Replace plastic water bottles and storage containers with glass or Pyrex glassware.

☐ Start the *Fat Loss Revolution* Phase 1 workouts.

☐ Perform one interval sprint workout. (p. 265)

☐ Write your scheduled time for exercise into your calendar.

☐ Throughout the day, stand more and sit less.

◈_____◈

## Week 4

☐ Continue with the checklist from the prior weeks.

☐ Continue with the Phase 1 workouts, A and B.

☐ Take your measurements and log them in your journal.

☐ Take updated photos.

☐ Continue with the checklist from the prior weeks.

☐ Perform one of the interval fat blaster – REV It Up workouts found on pages 246-261.

☐ Toss out toxic personal care products, household cleaning items, soaps, air fresheners, etc., and replace with non-toxic alternatives.

☐ Try one new vegetable or leafy green.

◈_____◈

## Week 5

- ☐ Continue with the checklist from the prior weeks.
- ☐ Take your measurements and log them in your journal.
- ☐ Take updated photos.
- ☐ Continue with Phase 1 workouts, A and B.
- ☐ Make and take your lunch to work versus eating out.
- ☐ Implement some of the detox solutions found in *Chapter 8*.
- ☐ Start your day with a green drink (see recipes in *Chapter 15*).
- ☐ Keep track of your workout progress in a journal.

◈_____◈

## Week 6

- ☐ Continue with the checklist from the prior weeks.
- ☐ Continue with Phase 1 workouts, A and B.
- ☐ Take your measurements and log them in your journal.
- ☐ Take updated photos.
- ☐ Invite supportive friends over for a healthy dinner or lunch.
- ☐ If you experience a setback, get right back on track.
- ☐ Schedule an appointment for annual blood work.

◈_____◈

## Week 7

- ☐ Continue with the checklist from the prior weeks.
- ☐ Take your measurements and log them in your journal.
- ☐ Take updated photos.
- ☐ Begin Phase 2 workouts.
- ☐ Take one full day off from intense exercise.
- ☐ Implement a relaxation-type activity into your schedule.
- ☐ Visualize yourself succeeding.

◈_____◈

## Week 8

- ☐ Continue with the checklist from the prior weeks.
- ☐ Continue with Phase 2 workouts, A and B.
- ☐ Take your measurements and log them in your journal.
- ☐ Take updated photos.
- ☐ Try a new type of fish at one of your meals.
- ☐ Possibly opt for a workout partner.
- ☐ Review and update your goals.

◈_____◈

## Week 9

- ☐ Continue with the checklist from the prior weeks.
- ☐ Continue with Phase 2 workouts, A and B.
- ☐ Take your measurements and log them in your journal.
- ☐ Take updated photos.
- ☐ Review your food journal and workout logs.
- ☐ Make sure you're eating three solid meals daily that contain protein and fiber from vegetables and leafy greens.

◈_____◈

## Week 10

- ☐ Continue with the checklist from the prior weeks.
- ☐ Continue with Phase 2 workouts, A and B.
- ☐ Take your measurements and log them in your journal.
- ☐ Take updated photos.
- ☐ Empower and inspire others by sharing your new fat loss lifestyle.

◈_____◈

## Week 11

- ☐ Continue with the checklist from the prior weeks.
- ☐ Start Phase 3 workouts.
- ☐ Take your measurements and log them in your journal.
- ☐ Take updated photos.

◆————————————————————————◆

## Week 12

- ☐ Continue with the checklist from the prior weeks.
- ☐ Continue Phase 3 workouts, A and B.
- ☐ Take your measurements and log them in your journal.
- ☐ Take updated photos.
- ☐ Review and update your goals, if needed.

◆————————————————————————◆

## Celebrate Your Personal *Fat Loss Revolution*

Congratulations on finishing the 12 week *Fat Loss Revolution*. Now it's time to celebrate your success and your hot 'n healthy body.

- ☐ Continue with the checklists from the prior weeks.
- ☐ Buy yourself a new outfit.
- ☐ Spend the day at a resort or spa for some well-deserved pampering.
- ☐ Send your success story to your local newspaper.
- ☐ Make a charitable contribution and donate your fat clothes to your favorite charity because you have no intention of ever wearing them again!
- ☐ Continue your *Fat Loss Revolution* as a lifestyle.

◆————————————————————————◆

# FINAL WORDS

Thank you for reading the *Fat Loss Revolution*. I invite you to return to the pages of this book again and again to re-energize and motivate yourself. You will gain more insight and value each time you read and review the information covered in this book.

Remember, optimal health and fat loss is a journey, a process and a lifestyle. Having a solid plan to direct you encourages a positive and successful outcome.

I would love to hear about your 12-week *Fat Loss Revolution* journey and your transformation. Please visit PaulaOwens.com to share your personal success story.

Be sure to visit my blog, http://thepowerof4-paula.blogspot.com, and my website, www.PaulaOwens.com, to get your free weekly wellness videos and free newsletters.

*From my heart to yours* ♥

*All my best to you, with love,*

*Paula Owens*

> *Fat loss is a process and a journey for a lifetime.*
>
> *Knowledge, balance and consistency are the keys to a Hot 'n Healthy Body at Any Age.*
>
> *You now have the information and the no-fail solutions for your personal Fat Loss Revolution.*

# RESOURCES AND RECOMMENDATIONS

*Supplements, protein powder, vitamins, exercise equipment,*
*recipe books, one-on-one consultations*
www.PaulaOwens.com

❖_____❖

*Environmental Working Group*
www.ewg.org

❖_____❖

*Grass-fed beef*
www.GrasslandBeef.com

❖_____❖

*Harpenden skinfold calipers*
www.harpenden-skinfold.com

❖_____❖

*Smart Seafood Guide*
www.foodandwaterwatch.org

❖_____❖

# ACKNOWLEDGEMENTS

I express my heartfelt gratitude and genuine appreciation to everyone who supported me throughout the process of this book.

Love and admiration to my Mother, my biggest fan, for her ongoing encouragement and instilling within me the four magical Ds – drive, dedication, desire and discipline.

I extend respect and recognition to all of my past, present and future teachers that have been a part of my life.

Gratitude and sincere thanks to my awesome editor, Diane Stevens, of Creative Pen & Mic.

Thank you to the incredibly gifted and very talented artist, Charlie Aligaen, for his amazing drawings of the exercise illustrations.

Thank you to my dear friend, Maria DePasquale, for proofreading the *Fat Loss Revolution* manuscript and for your recipe contributions.

Thank you to my sweet friend and primal nutritionist, Cate Munroe of Cate's Nutrition Kitchen, for your delicious recipe contributions.

Thanks to fitness model, Rebecca Rausch, for modeling the exercise illustrations. Yours truly was also one of the fitness models.

Thank you, NetPub, for your creative cover design.

Thank you to my Higher Power, God, and to you – the readers, my siblings, clients, colleagues and dear friends.

*With love, appreciation and gratitude,* ♥

*Paula Owens*

# REFERENCES

## Introduction

Chapman, C.D., et al. (2012). Lifestyle determinants of the drive to eat: a meta-analysis. *American Journal of Clinical Nutrition, 96*(3), 492-97.

## Chapter 1

Huffman, M. U. S. population on track to getting even fatter. (2011, November 17). *ScienceDaily*. Retrieved from http://www.sciencedaily.com/releases/2011/11/111116132920.htm

Guidelines for Exercise Testing and Prescription, 6th edition. (2000). American College of Sports Medicine.

Resource Manual for Guidelines for Exercise Testing and Prescription, 4th Ed. (2001). American College of Sports Medicine.

Muth, N.D. What are the guidelines for percentage of body fat loss? (2009, December 2). *American Council on Exercise*. Retrieved from http://www.acefitness.org/blog/112/what-are-the-guidelines-for-percentage-of-body-fat?

## Chapter 2

Poliquin, C. (2011, March). *Poliquin Performance*. Presentation delivered at *Biosignature certification course,* Scottsdale, AZ.

Henry, B., & Clarke, I. (2008). Research adds weight to fat burning theories. Department of Physiology in the Faculty of Medicine, Nursing and Health Sciences, Monash University, Melbourne, Australia. Retrieved from http://www.monash.edu.au/news/releases/show/1047

Rosmond, R., et al. (1998). Stress-related cortisol secretion in men: relationships with abdominal obesity and endocrine, metabolic, and hemodynamic abnormalities. *Journal of Clinical Endocrinology and Metabolism, 83*, 1853-59.

Patrick, L. (2009). Thyroid disruption: Mechanisms and clinical implications in human health. *Alternative Medicine Review, 14*(4), 326-46.

Meeker, J., et al. (2007). Di(2-ethylhexyl) phthalate metabolites may alter thyroid hormone levels in men. *Environmental Health Perspectives, 115*(7), 1029-34.

Souza, L. L., et al. (2010). Effects of dietary fish oil on thyroid hormone signaling in the liver. *Journal of Nutritional Biochemistry, 21*(10), 935-40.

Blom, W., et al. (2006). Effect of a high-protein breakfast on the postprandial ghrelin response. *American Journal of Clinical Nutrition, 83*(2), 211-20.

Rask, E., et al. (2012). Cortisol metabolism after weight loss - associations with 11 β-hsd type 1 and markers of obesity in women. *Clinical Endocrinology.*

Kravitz, L. et al. (n.d.). Cortisol connection: Tips on managing stress and weight. University of New Mexico, Albuquerque, NM. Retrieved from http://www.unm.edu/~lkravitz/Article%20folder/stresscortisol.html

Taheri, S., et al. (2004). Short sleep duration is associated with reduced leptin, elevated ghrelin, and increased body mass index. *PLoS Medicine, 1*(3). Retrieved from http://www.plosmedicine.org/article/info%3Adoi%2F10.1371%2Fjournal.pmed.0010062.

Dirlewanger, M., et al. (2000). Effects of short-term carbohydrate or fat overfeeding on energy expenditure and plasma leptin concentrations in healthy female subjects. *International Journal of Obesity and Related Metabolism Disorders, 24*(11), 1413-18.

Cnop, M., et al. (2002). The concurrent accumulation of intra-abdominal and subcutaneous fat explains the association between insulin resistance and plasma leptin concentrations: Distinct metabolic effects of two fat compartments. *Diabetes, 51*(4), 1005-15.

Yamauchi, T., et al. (2001). The fat-derived hormone adiponectin reverses insulin resistance associated with both lipoatrophy and obesity. *Nature Medicine, 7*(8), 941-46.

Fragopoulou, E., et al. (2010). The association between adherence to the Mediterranean Diet and adiponectin levels among healthy adults: the Attica study. *Journal of Nutritional Biochemistry, 21*(4), 285-89.

**Chapter 3**

Akiko, N. (2010). Rice intake and type 2 diabetes in Japanese men and women: the Japan Public Health Center–based Prospective Study. *American Journal of Clinical Nutrition, 92*, 1468-77.

Alvarez, J. A. (2010). Serum 25-hydroxyvitamin d and parathyroid hormone are independent determinants of whole-body insulin sensitivity in women and may contribute to lower insulin sensitivity in african americans. *American Journal of Clinical Nutrition, 92*, 1344-49.

Mekary, R. (2012). Eating patterns and type 2 diabetes risk in men: breakfast omission, eating frequency, and snacking. *American Journal of Clinical Nutrition*, *95*, 1182-89.

McEwen, B. S. (1980). The brain as a target of endocrine hormones. *Neuroendocrinology*, 33-42. Krieger and Hughes, Eds.

Mariemi, J. (2002). Visceral fat and psychosocial stress in identical twins discordant for obesity. *Journal of Internal Medicine*, *251*, 35-43.

Schwarzbein, D. (2004). *The Schwarzbein principle: the program: losing weight the healthy way*. Deerfield Beach, FL: Health Communications. Heymsfield, S. B., et al. (1995). The calorie: Myth, measurement and reality. *American Journal of Clinical Nutrition*, *62*, 1034-41.

Nickols-Richardson, S. M., et al. (2005). Perceived hunger is lower and weight loss is greater in overweight pre-menopausal women consuming a low-carbohydrate/high-protein vs. high-carbohydrate/low-fat diet. *Journal of the American Dietetic Association*, *105*(9), 1433-37.

Manninen, A. H. (2004). Is a calorie really a calorie? *Journal of the International Society of Sports Nutrition*, *1*(2), 21-26.

Feinman, R. D., & Fine, E. J. (2004). A calorie is a calorie" violates the second law of thermodynamics. *Nutrition Journal*, *3*(9)

Howarth, N. C., et al. (2001). Dietary fiber and weight regulation. *Nutrition Review*, *59*(5), 129-39.

Wardlaw, G. M., & Kessel, M. (2002). *Perspectives in nutrition*. (2nd ed., pp. 535-37). New York, NY: McGraw-Hill Higher Education.

Jéquier, E. (2002). Pathways to obesity. *International Journal of Obesity and Related Metabolic Disorders*, *26*(2), 12-17.

Mekary, R. A., et al. (2012). Eating patterns and type 2 diabetes risk in men: breakfast omission, eating frequency, and snacking. *American Journal of Clinical Nutrition*, *95*(5), 1182-89. Retrieved from http://www.ajcn.org/content/95/5/1182.abstract?etoc

Hoyland, A., et al. (2009). A systematic review of the effect of breakfast on the cognitive performance of children and adolescents. *Nutrition Research Reviews*, *22*(2), 220-43.

Wansink, B., et al. (2012). First foods most: After 18-hour fast, people drawn to starches first and vegetables last. *Archives of Internal Medicine*, *172*(12), 961-63.

Kong, A., et al. (2012). Self-monitoring and eating-related behaviors are associated with 12-month weight loss in postmenopausal overweight-to-obese women. *Journal of the Academy of Nutrition and Dietetics, 112*(9), 1428-35.

Cereda, E., et al. (2011). Weight cycling is associated with body weight excess and abdominal fat accumulation: A cross-sectional study. *Clinical Nutrition, 30*(6), 718-23.

Yunsheng, M., et al. (2003). Association between eating patterns and obesity in a free-living US adult population. *American Journal of Epidemiology, 158*(1), 85-92.

Mhurchu, C. N., et al. (2010). Effects of a free school breakfast programme on school attendance, achievement, psychosocial function, and nutrition: a stepped wedge cluster randomised trial. *BMC Public Health, 10*, 738. Retrieved from http://www.biomedcentral.com/1471-2458/10/738

Farshchi, H. R., et al. (2005). Deleterious effects of omitting breakfast on insulin sensitivity and fasting lipid profiles in healthy lean women. *The American Journal of Clinical Nutrition, 81*(2), 388-96.

Kartashov, A. I. (2003, March 6). *Eurekalert: Eating breakfast may reduce risk of obesity, diabetes, heart disease.* American Heart Association Conference on Cardiovascular Disease Epidemiology and Prevention, Miami, FL.

Bazzano, L. A., et al. (2005). Dietary intake of whole and refined grain breakfast cereals and weight gain in men. *Obesity Research, 13*(11), 1952-60. Retrieved from http://www.ncbi.nlm.nih.gov/pubmed/16339127

Mori, A. M., et al. (2011). Acute and second-meal effects of almond form in impaired glucose tolerant adults: a randomized crossover trial. *Nutrition & Metabolism, 8*(6). Retrieved from http://www.nutritionandmetabolism.com/content/8/1/6

**Chapter 4**

Aeberli, I., et al. (2011). Low to moderate sugar-sweetened beverage consumption impairs glucose and lipid metabolism and promotes inflammation in healthy young men: a randomized controlled trial. *American Journal of Clinical Nutrition, 94*(2), 479-85.

Mozaffarian, D., et al. (2004). Dietary intake of trans fatty acids and systemic inflammation in women. *American Journal of Clinical Nutrition, 79*(4), 606.

Grzanna, R., et al. (2005). Ginger – an herbal medicinal product with broad anti-inflammatory actions. *Journal of Medicinal Food, 8*(2), 125-32.

Jang, S., et al. (2010). Luteolin inhibits microglia and alters hippocampal-dependent spatial working memory in aged mice. *Journal of Nutrition, 140*(10), 1892-98

Chacko, S. A., et al. (2010). Relations of dietary magnesium intake to biomarkers of inflammation and endothelial dysfunction in an ethnically diverse cohort of postmenopausal women. *Diabetes Care, 33*(2), 304-10. Retrieved from http://www.wellnessresources.com/studies/entry/magnesium_is_needed_to_reduce_inflammation

Sharman, M. J., & Volek, J. S. (2004). Weight loss leads to reductions in inflammatory biomarkers after a very-low-carbohydrate diet and a low-fat diet in overweight men. *Clinical Science, 107*(4), 365-69.

Simpson, N., & Dinges, D. F. (2007). Sleep and inflammation. *Nutrition Reviews, 65*(1), 244-52.

American Academy of Sleep Medicine (2009). Inflammation may be link between extreme sleep durations and poor health. *ScienceDaily.* Retrieved from http://www.sciencedaily.com /releases/2009/02/090201094119.htm

O'Hara, A. M., & Shanahan, F. (2006). The gut flora as a forgotten organ. *EMBO Reports, 7*(7), 688-93.

Ley, R. E. (2006). Microbial ecology: human gut microbes associated with obesity. *Nature, 444*(7122), 1022-23.

Turnbaugh, P. J., et al. (2006). An obesity-associated gut microbiome with increased capacity for energy harvest. *Nature, 444*(7122), 1027-31.

Messaoudi, M., et al. (2010). Assessment of psychotropic-like properties of a probiotic formulation (lactobacillus helveticus r0052 and bifidobacterium longum r0175) in rats and humans. *British Journal of Nutrition,* 1-9.

Delzenne, N. M., & Cani, P. D. (2010). Nutritional modulation of gut microbiota in the context of obesity and insulin resistance: Potential interest of prebiotics. *International Dairy Journal, 20*(4), 277-80.

Kdooka, Y., et al. (2010). Regulation of abdominal adiposity by probiotics (lactobacillus gasseri sbt2055) in adults with obese tendencies in a randomized controlled trial. *European Journal of Clinical Nutrition, 64,* 636-43.

Collado, M. C., et al. (2009). The impact of probiotic on gut health. *Current Drug Metabolism, 10*(1), 68-78.

**Chapter 5**

Reichert, B., et al. (2011). Concerted action of aldehyde dehydrogenases influences depot-specific fat formation. *Molecular Endocrinology, 25*(5), 799-809.

Irving, B. A., et al. (2008). Effect of exercise training intensity on abdominal visceral fat and body composition. *Medicine Science Sports Exercise, 22*(6), 2036-44.

Yamamoto, L. M., et al. (2008). The effects of resistance training on endurance distance running performance among highly trained runners: A systematic review. *The Journal of Strength and Conditioning Research, 22*(6), 2036-44.

Assuncao, M. L., et al. (2009). Effects of dietary coconut oil on the biochemical and anthropometric profiles of women presenting abdominal obesity. *Lipids, 44*(7), 593-601.

Wake Forest Baptist Medical Center (2011). Soluble fiber strikes a blow to belly fat. *ScienceDaily*. Retrieved from http://www.sciencedaily.com/releases/2011/06/110627123032.htm

Hamburger, R. (1982). Proceedings of the First International Symposium on Food Allergy, Vancouver, B.C.

Perelmutter, L. (1984). Non-IgE mediated atopic disease. *Annals of Allergy, Asthma and Immunology, 52*, 640-68.

Ebbeling, C. B., et al. (2004). Compensation for energy intake from fast food among overweight and lean adolescents. *Journal of the American Medical Association, 291*(23), 2828-33.

Brownell, K. D., et al. (2010). Personal responsibility and obesity: A constructive approach to a controversial issue. *Health Affairs (Millwood), 29*(3), 379-87.

Daniells, S. (2009). Green tea may ease mental distress: Study. *Bergstrom Nutrition*. Retrieved from http://www.nutraingredients-usa.com/Research/Green-tea-may-ease-mental-distress-Study

Epel, E., et al. (2001). Stress may add bite to appetite in women: a laboratory study of stress-induced cortisol and eating behavior. *Psychoneuroendocrinology, 26*(1), 37-49.

Maldonado, M. D., et al. (2012). Melatonin administrated immediately before an intense exercise reverses oxidative stress, improves immunological defenses and lipid metabolism in football players. *Physiology & Behavior, 105*(5), 1099-1103.

Martin, F. J., et al. (2009). Metabolic effects of dark chocolate consumption on energy, gut microbiota, and stress-related metabolism in free-living subjects. *Journal of Proteome Research, 8*(12), 5568-79.

Hatori, M., et al. (2012). Time-restricted feeding without reducing caloric intake prevents metabolic diseases in mice fed a high-fat diet. *Cell Metabolism, 15*(6), 848-60.

Nedeltcheva, A.V., et al., (2010). Insufficient sleep undermines dietary efforts to reduce adiposity. *Annals of Internal Medicine*, 153(7):435-441.

Broussard, J.L., et al. (2012). Impaired insulin signaling in human adipocytes after experimental sleep restriction. *Annals of Internal Medicine*, 157(8):549-557

Watson, N. F., et al. (2012). Sleep duration and body mass index in twins: a gene-environment interaction. *Sleep, 35*(5), 597-603.

## Chapter 6

Edling, L., et al. (2012). Celiac disease and giardiasis: a case report. *European Journal of Gastroenterology & Hepatology, 24*(8), 984-87.

Lipski, E. (2000). *Digestive Wellness.* (2nd ed.). Lincolnwood, IL: Keats Publishing.

Eidenier, H. O. (2011). *Acid-base balance and hypochlorhydria.* Presentation delivered at Blood chemistry analysis seminar, Scottsdale, AZ.

Wright, J., & Lenard, L. (2001). *Why stomach acid is good for you.* Lanham, MD: M. Evans & Co., Inc.

Kadooka, Y. E. A. (2010). Regulation of abdominal adiposity by probiotics (lactobacillus gasseri sbt2055) in adults with obese tendencies in a randomized controlled trial. *European Journal of Clinical Nutrition, 64,* 636-43.

## Chapter 7

Freed, D. L. (1999). Do dietary lectins cause disease? *British Medical Journal, 318*(7190), 1023-24.

Courdain, L. (1999). Cereal grains: Humanity's double-edged sword. *World Review of Nutrition and Dietetics, 84,* 19-73.

Conventional vs. organic: It's not about getting more, but getting less for your money. Less pesticides, dioxins & co. (2012, Sept 7). *SuppVersity.* Retrieved from http://suppversity.blogspot.com/2012/09/conventional-vs-organic-its-not-about.html

Biesiekierski, J. R., et al. (2011). Gluten causes gastrointestinal symptoms in subjects without celiac disease: A double-blind randomized placebo-controlled trial. *American Journal of Gastroenterology, 106*(3), 508-14.

Bernal, S. Y., et al. (2010). Opioid receptor antagonism in the nucleus accumbens fails to block the expression of sugar-conditioned flavor preferences in rats. *Pharmacology Biochemistry and Behavior, 95*(1), 56-62.

McCann, D., et al. (2007). Food additives and hyperactive behaviour in 3-year-old and 8/9-year-old children in the community: a randomised, double-blinded, placebo-controlled trial. *The Lancet, 370*(9598), 1560-67.

American Chemical Society (2007, August 23). Soda warning? High-fructose corn syrup linked to diabetes, new study suggests. *ScienceDaily.* Retrieved from http://www.sciencedaily.com /releases/2007/08/070823094819.htm

Blaylock, R. L. (1997). *Excitotoxins: The taste that kills.* Santa Fe, NM: Health Press.

University of Barcelona (2007, March 16). Fructose-sweetened beverages increases risk of obesity in rats. *ScienceDaily.* Retrieved from http://www.sciencedaily.com /releases/2007/03/070315123558.htm

American Psychological Association (2008, February 11). Artificial sweeteners linked to weight gain. *ScienceDaily.* Retrieved from http://www.sciencedaily.com /releases/2008/02/080210183902.htm

Kavanagh, K., et al. (2007). Trans fat diet induces abdominal obesity and changes in insulin sensitivity in monkeys. *Journal of Obesity, 15*(7), 1675-84.

Ostman, E. M., et al. (2001). Inconsistency between glycemic and insulemic responses to regular and fermented milk products. *American Journal of Clinical Nutrition, 74*(1), 96-100.

Daniel, K. (2005). *The whole soy story.* Washington, DC: Newtrends Publishing, Inc.

Hoppe, C., et al. (2005). High intakes of milk, but not meat, increases insulin and insulin resistance in 8-year-old boys. *European Journal of Clinical Nutrition, 59*(3), 393-98.

Genkinger, J. M., et al. (2006). Dairy products and ovarian cancer: a pooled analysis of 12 cohort studies. *Cancer Epidemiology Biomarkers Preview, 15*(2), 364-72.

Ganmaa, D., & Sato, A. (2005). The possible role of female sex hormones in milk from pregnant cows in the development of breast, ovarian, and corpus uteri cancers. *Medical Hypotheses, 65*, 1028-37.

Owusu, W., et al. (1997). Calcium intake and the incidence of forearm and hip fractures among men. *Journal of Nutrition, 127*, 1782-87.

Feskanich, D., et al. (1997). Milk, dietary calcium, and bone fractures in women: a 12-year prospective study. *American Journal of Public Health, 87*, 992-97.

Newbold, R. R., et al. (2008). Effects of endocrine disruptors on obesity. *Internal Journal of Andrology, 31*(2), 201-08.

Meeker, J. D., et al. (2010). Urinary bisphenol a concentrations in relation to serum thyroid and reproductive hormone levels in men from an infertility clinic. *Environmental Science & Technology, 44*(4), 1458-63.

Diamanti-Kandarakis, E., et al. (2009). Endocrine disrupting chemicals. An endocrine society scientific statement. *Endocrine Reviews, 30*(4), 293-342.

Beadle, L. (2010, February 26). List of xenoestrogens - chemical estrogens: How to avoid xenoestrogens. *Suite 101*. Retrieved from http://www.suite101.com/content/list-of-xenoestrogens---chemical-estrogens-a205523

University of California, Los Angeles (2012, May 15). This is your brain on sugar: Study shows high-fructose diet sabotages learning, memory. *ScienceDaily*. Retrieved from http://www.sciencedaily.com-/releases/2012/05/120515150938.htm

Wild, D. E. A. (2010). Evidence of high sugar intake, and low fibre and mineral intake, in the gluten-free diet. *Alimentary Pharmacology & Therapeutics Journal, 32*(4), 573-81.

Raloff, J. (2012). Tricks foods play. *Science News. 182*(7), 24.

## Chapter 8

Davis, D.L., et al. (1993). Medical Hypothesis: Xenoestrogens as Preventable Causes of Breast Cancer. *Environmental Health Perspectives,* 101:372-377.

Kozak, A., & Fought, A. (2011). Beyond alcohol and drug addiction. Does the negative trait of low distress tolerance have an association with overeating? *Appetite, 57*(3), 578-81.

Ibarluzea, J., et al. (2004). *Cancer Causes Control, 15*(6):591-600.

Nobel Foundation (2009, October 5). Telomere copy protection: Nobel goes to scientists who solved how chromosome ends work. (2009, Oct 5). *ScienceDaily,* Retrieved from http://www.sciencedaily.com-/releases/2009/10/091005110401.htm

Nedeltcheva, A. V., et al. (2010). Insufficient sleep undermines dietary efforts to reduce adiposity. *Annals of Internal Medicine, 153*(7), 435-41.

Morselli, L., et al. (2010). Role of sleep duration in the regulation of glucose metabolism and appetite. *Best Practice & Research: Clinical Endocrinology & Metabolism, 24*(5), 687-702.

Vgontzas, A. N., et al. (2001). Chronic insomnia is associated with nyctohemeral activation of the hypothalamic-pituitary-adrenal axis: Clinical implications. *Journal of Clinical Endocrinology & Metabolism, 86*(8), 3787-94.

Hatori, M., et al. (2012). Time-restricted feeding without reducing caloric intake prevents metabolic diseases in mice fed a high-fat diet. *Cell Metabolism, 15*(6), 848-60.

## Chapter 9

Logel, C., et al. (2011). The role of the self in physical health: Testing the effect of a values-affirmation intervention on weight loss. *Psychological Science, 23*(1), 53-55.

Johnston, C. S., et al. (2004). Vinegar improves insulin sensitivity to a high-carbohydrate meal in subjects with insulin resistance or type 2 diabetes. *Diabetes Care, 27*(1), 281-82.

Vlassara, H., et al. (2002). Inflammatory mediators are induced by dietary glycotoxins, a major risk factor for diabetic angiopathy. *Proceedings of the National Academy of Sciences USA, 99*(24), 15596-15601.

Johnston, C. S., et al. (2010). Examination of the antiglycemic properties of vinegar in healthy adults. *Annals of Nutrition & Metabolism, 56*(1), 74-79.

Li, J., et al. (2011). Improvement in chewing activity reduces energy intake in one meal and modulates plasma gut hormone concentrations in obese and lean young Chinese men. *American Journal of Clinical Nutrition, 94*(3), 709-16.

European Society of Endocrinology. (2012, May 06). Eating fast increases diabetes risk. *ScienceDaily*. Retrieved from http://www.sciencedaily.com /releases/2012/05/120507210038.htm

Siler, S. Q., et al. (1999). Denovo lipogenesis, lipid kinetics and whole-body lipid balances in humans after acute alcohol consumption. *American Journal of Clinical Nutrition, 70*(5), 928-36.

van Ittersum, K., & Wansink, B. (2012). Plate size and color suggestibility: the Delboeuf illusion's bias on serving and eating behavior. *Journal of Consumer Research*, Retrieved from http://www.jstor.org/stable/10.1086/662615

Brandhagen, M., et al. (2012). Alcohol and macronutrient intake patterns are related to general and central adiposity. *European Journal of Clinical Nutrition , 66*, 305-13.

**Chapter 11**

Talanian, J. L., et al. (2007). Two weeks of high-intensity aerobic interval training increases the capacity for fat oxidation during exercise in women. *Journal of Applied Physiology, 102*(4), 1439-47.

Irving, B. A., et al. (2008). Effect of exercise training intensity on abdominal visceral fat and body composition. *Medicine and Science in Sports and Exercise, 40*(11), 1863-72.

ACSM. (1998). *ACSM's resource manual for guidelines for exercise testing and prescription*. (3rd ed.). Philadelphia, PA: Lippincott Williams & Wilkins.

Anon. (2008). Whey protein. *Alternative Medicine Review, 13*(4), 342-49.
Hayes, A., & Cribb, P. J. (2008). Effect of whey protein isolate on strength, body composition and muscle hypertrophy during resistance training. *Current Opinion in Clinical Nutrition & Metabolic Care. 11*(1), 40-44.

Acheson, K. J., et al. (2011). Protein choices targeting thermogenesis and metabolism. *American Journal of Clinical Nutrition, 93*(3), 525-34.

Hackney, K. J. (2010). Timing protein intake increases energy expenditure 24 h after resistance training. *Medicine and Science in Sports and Exercise, 42*(5), 998-1003.

Heydari, M. et al. (2012). The effect of high-intensity intermittent exercise on body composition of overweight young males. *Journal of Obesity, 2012,* 480467.

Boutcher, S. H. (2011). High-intensity intermittent exercise and fat loss. *Journal of Obesity, 2011,* 868305.

Stookey, J. D., et al. (2012). Orange juice limits postprandial fat oxidation after breakfast in normal-weight adolescents and adults. *Advances in Nutrition, 3*(4), 629S-35S.

Watford, M., & Wu, G. (2011). Protein. *Advances in Nutrition, 2,* 62-63.

Scott, C. B., & Kemp, R. B. (2005). direct and indirect calorimetry of lactate oxidation: Implications for whole-body energy expenditure. *Journal of Sports Sciences, 23*(1), 15-19.

Newsom, S. A., et al. (2010). Energy deficit after exercise augments lipid mobilization but does not contribute to the exercise-induced increase in insulin sensitivity. *Journal of Applied Physiology, 108*(3), 554-60.

Churchward-Venne, T. A., et al. (2012). Nutritional regulation of muscle protein synthesis with resistance exercise: strategies to enhance anabolism. *Nutrition & Metabolism, 9,* 40.

Talanian, J. L., et al. (2007). Two weeks of high-intensity aerobic interval training increases the capacity for fat oxidation during exercise in women. *Journal of Applied Physiology, 102*(4), 1439-47.

Burgomaster, K. A., et al. (2008). Similar metabolic adaptations during exercise after low volume sprint interval and traditional endurance training in humans. *Journal of Physiology, 586*(1), 151-60.

Hazell, T. J., et al. (2012). Two minutes of sprint-interval exercise elicits 24-hr oxygen consumption similar to that of 30 min of continuous endurance exercise. *International Journal of Sport Nutrition and Exercise Metabolism, 22*(4), 276-83.

Bryner, R. W., et al. (1999). Effects of resistance vs. aerobic training combined with an 800 calorie liquid diet on lean body mass and resting metabolic rate. *Journal of the American College of Nutrition, 18*(2), 115-21.

American Heart Association. (2012, March 14). Walking may lessen the influence of genes on obesity by half. *ScienceDaily*, Retrieved from http://www.sciencedaily.com /releases/2012/03/120314142833.htm

## Chapter 12

Li, Y., et al. (2010). Effects of multivitamin and mineral supplementation on adiposity, energy expenditure and lipid profiles in obese Chinese women. *International Journal of Obesity (London), 34*(6), 1070-77.

Fletcher, R.H., & Fairfield, K.M. (2002). Vitamins for chronic disease prevention in adults. *Journal of the American Medical Association, 287*(23), 3127–29.

## Chapter 13

Wansink, B., et al. (2012). First foods most: After 18-hour fast, people drawn to starches first and vegetables last. *Archives of Internal Medicine, 172*(12), 961-63.
Karst, H., et al. (1984). Diet-induced thermogenesis in man: thermic effects of single proteins, carbohydrates and fats depending on their energy amount. *Annals of Nutrition and Metabolism, 28*, 245-52.

Johnston, C. S. (2005). Strategies for healthy weight loss: From vitamin C to the glycemic response. *Journal of the American College of Nutrition, 24*(3), 158-65.

Daley, C. A. (2010). A review of fatty acid profiles and antioxidant content in grass-fed and grain-fed beef. *Nutrition Journal, 9*, 10.

Castellini, C., et al. (2002). Effect of organic production system on broiler carcass and meat quality. *Meat Science, 60*(3), 219-25.

Pal, S., et al. (2010). Effects of whey protein isolate on body composition, lipids, insulin and glucose in overweight and obese individuals. *British Journal of Nutrition, 104*(5), 716-23.

Kong, A., et al. (2012). Self-monitoring and eating-related behaviors associated with 12-month weight loss among postmenopausal overweight-to-obese women in a dietary weight loss intervention. *Journal of the Academy of Nutrition and Dietetics, 112*(9), 1428-35.

Harvard Medical School. (2004, August). Coffee health risks: For the moderate drinker, coffee is safe says Harvard Women's Health Watch. *Harvard Health Publications*. Retrieved from http://www.health.harvard.edu/press_releases/coffee_health_risk

Anon. (2012, January 4). CLA reduced body fat in overweight children. *Health Studies Journal*. Retrieved from http://www.nhiondemand.com/hsjarticle.aspx?id=947

Binnert, C., et al. (1998). Influence of human obesity on the metabolic fate of dietary long- and medium-chain triacylglycerols. *American Journal of Clinical Nutrition, 67*(4), 595-601.

Fife, B. (2005). *Coconut cures: Preventing and treating common health problems with coconut*. Colorado Springs, CO: Piccadilly Books, Ltd. Assunção, M. L., et al. (2009). Effects of dietary coconut oil on the biochemical and anthropometric profiles of women presenting abdominal obesity. *Lipids, 44*(7), 593-601.

Lejeune, M., et al. (2003). Effect of capsaicin on substrate oxidation and weight maintenance after modest body-weight loss in human subjects. *British Journal of Nutrition, 90*(3), 651.

Tomoo, K., et al. (2009). Acetic acid upregulates the expression of genes for fatty acid oxidation enzymes in liver to suppress body fat accumulation. *Journal of Agricultural Food Chemistry, 57*(13), 5982-86.

Tang, Q., et al. (2008). Fluoride and children's intelligence: a meta-analysis. *Biological Trace Element Research, 126*(1-3), 115-20.

Reinbach, H. C. (2009). Effects of capsaicin, green tea and ch-19 sweet pepper on appetite and energy intake in humans in negative and positive energy balance. *Clinical Nutrition, 28*(3), 260-65.

Kondo, T., et al. (2009). Acetic acid upregulates the expression of genes for fatty acid oxidation enzymes in liver to suppress body fat accumulation. *Journal of Agricultural and Food Chemistry, 57*(13), 5982-86.

Goltz, S. R., et al. (2012). Meal triacylglycerol profile modulates postprandial absorption of carotenoids in humans. *Molecular Nutrition & Food Research, 56*(6), 866-77.

**Chapter 14**

Fred Hutchinson Cancer Research Center. (2012, July 13). Want to lose weight? Keep a food journal, don't skip meals and avoid going out to lunch. *ScienceDaily*, Retrieved from http://www.sciencedaily.com-/releases/2012/07/120713080029.htm

Stookey, J. D., et al. (2012). Orange juice limits postprandial fat oxidation after breakfast in normal-weight adolescents and adults. *Advances in Nutrition, 3*(4), 629S-35S.

# INDEX

## A

alcohol  15, 31, 42, 66, 84, 89, 91-92, 106, 135, 156-157, 159-164, 167

addictions  158-165

adiponectin  38

adrenal  22-23, 25-30, 42, 47, 70, 75, 79, 83-85, 160, 162, 172, 267

AGEs 118, 155-156

andregenic, beta and alpha  31

anti-nutrient  113

anxiety  27, 71-72, 74, 76, 86, 89, 164

artificial sweeteners  49, 55, 66, 112, 118, 123-124, 130, 135, 164, 176, 274, 299,   302

## B

bacteria  72, 89-92, 97-98, 123, 128, 133, 282

belly fat  17-18, 27, 38, 61-53, 66, 72, 81, 90, 97, 114, 116, 145, 157, 169, 172, 263

Biosignature 11

blood sugar  16-19, 26-26, 45-46, 48-50, 52, 57, 61, 71, 74, 83, 114, 116-118, 124, 132, 135, 145, 160, 162-163, 171, 277, 284-285, 287, 290

body fat  5-6, 8-12, 15, 17, 28, 37-38, 43-44, 47, 52, 54, 55, 61, 64-65, 69, 71, 80-81, 89, 94, 107, 118, 121, 124, 131, 144, 170, 263, 277

BPA  18, 33, 109

breakfast  36, 47-52, 136, 162, 292-294

## C

calories  10, 36-37, 43-46, 52, 115, 121, 153, 173, 179

Candida  25, 42, 58, 72, 90, 92, 94, 99, 107, 114, 132-133, 160, 284

carbohydrates  17-20, 23, 36, 43-46, 53, 55-56, 63, 71, 116, 123, 144-145, 150, 153, 159-160, 164, 278 cardio  28, 42, 171, 180, 263

coconut oil  56, 62, 92-93, 125, 154, 163, 283-284

coffee  20, 49, 110, 118, 178, 289, 291-292

cortisol  22, 26-30, 37, 39, 44, 54, 59, 62-63, 66, 70-71, 73, 75, 77-
78, 81, 83-84,  87, 90, 97, 103, 139, 157, 160, 172, 263,
268-269, 287, 289

cravings  15, 28, 46, 49, 72, 81, 115, 118, 123-124, 142, 157-166,
272, 277, 284,  290, 292

# D

dairy  66, 83, 92, 99, 102-103, 110, 112-113, 119-120

detox  35, 63, 109, 131-139, 276, 287

diabetes  4, 17-18, 33, 47, 53, 59, 114, 117, 121, 124, 126, 289

digestion  78, 89-100,  134, 148, 152, 275, 287, 290

# E

Electromagnetic (EMF) 72, 78, 136

estrogen  30-35, 62, 65, 107-111, 118, 126-127, 133, 157

exercise  77, 82, 169-269

# F

fasting  27, 42, 85, 138

fiber  35, 46, 49, 61-62, 116, 135, 139, 145, 150, 163, 165, 276, 285-
286, 293

fish oil  20, 26, 275

food journal  55, 57, 67, 134, 145, 149

food sensitivity, intolerance, allergy  57, 6 4-68, 87, 90, 114-115,
161

frankenfats  101, 112, 126, 135, 300

frankenfood  101, 135, 158

# G

genetically-engineered  48, 101-102, 105, 118, 121, 127-128, 154,
158, 299-300

ghrelin  36, 44-46, 80, 115

supplements  59, 66, 92, 95, 99, 111, 139, 163, 165, 178, 271-276,
        282-283

# T

thyroid  21-26, 28, 32, 37, 42, 85-86, 107, 114, 121, 123, 126-127,
        132, 284, 289
toxins  84, 90-92, 103, 110, 127, 131-133, 280

# V

visceral  27-29, 37-38, 61, 63, 97, 103, 170, 263, 279, 282
vitamins  59, 66, 92, 95, 99, 111, 139, 163, 165, 178, 271-276, 282-
        283

# W

water  29, 51, 57, 74, 98, 110-111, 134, 152, 154, 175, 287-288
weight loss  9-10
workouts  169-269
wheat  23, 55, 66, 83, 92, 99, 112-117, 130, 132, 135, 164, 299-300

# X

xenoestrogens  32-33, 35, 108, 133, 285

## ABOUT THE AUTHOR

Paula Owens, M.S., is a Nutritionist, Certified Fitness Professional, Holistic Health Practitioner, and Fat Loss Expert. For over 20 years, Paula has worked with the most challenging weight loss resistant individuals to transform their bodies and lives, and she has led thousands of other people with a variety of health disorders to attain improved overall health, fitness, energy and well-being.

"I am passionate and dedicated to helping people achieve exceptional levels of health by educating and empowering them with cutting-edge information and solutions to prevent disease and look and feel their best ever."

Paula holds a Master's degree in Holistic Nutrition, a Bachelor's degree in Kinesiology, and numerous professional health and fitness certifications. Paula has a private practice in the Phoenix, Arizona area and consults with clients all over the world. She is a health, nutrition and fitness columnist for several national health publications, and the creator of "21 Days to a Leaner, Healthier You," an online exercise and fat loss program.

Paula is also the author of *The Power of 4 – Your Ultimate Guide Guaranteed to Change Your Body and Transform Your Life.*

**For more information, visit
www.PaulaOwens.com**